Immunochemistry

Other titles in the series

OUTLINE STUDIES IN BIOLOGY

Editors : Professor T.W. Goodwin, F.R.S., University of Liverpool
Professor J.M. Ashworth, University of Essex

Editors' Foreword

The student of biological science in his final years as an undergraduate and his first years as a postgraduate is expected to gain some familiarity with current research at the frontiers of his discipline. New research work is published in a perplexing diversity of publications and is inevitably concerned with the minutiae of the subject. The sheer number of research journals and papers also causes confusion and difficulties of assimilation. Review articles usually presuppose a background knowledge of the field and are inevitably rather restricted in scope. There is thus the need for short but authoritative introductions to those areas of modern biological research which are either not dealt with in standard introductory textbooks or are not dealt with in sufficient detail to enable the student to go on from them to read scholarly reviews with profit. This series of books is designed to satisfy this need.

The authors have been asked to produce a brief outline of their subject assuming that their readers will have read and remembered much of a standard introductory textbook of biology. This outline then sets out to provide by building on this basis, the conceptual framework within which modern research work is progressing and aims to give the reader an indication of the problems, both conceptual and practical, which must be overcome if progress is to be maintained. We hope that students will go on to read the more detailed reviews and articles to which reference is made with a greater insight and understanding of how they fit into the overall scheme of modern research effort and may thus be helped to choose where to make their own contribution to this effort.

These books are guidebooks, not textbooks. Modern research pays scant regard for the academic divisions into which biological teaching and introductory textbooks must, to a certain extent, be divided. We have thus concentrated in this series on providing guides to those areas which fall between, or which involve, several different academic disciplines. It is here that the gap between the textbook and the research paper is widest and where the need for guidance is greatest. In so doing we hope to have extended or supplemented but not supplanted main texts and to have given students assistance in seeing how modern biological research is progressing while at the same time providing a foundation for self help in the achievement of successful examination results.

Immunochemistry

M.W. Steward
Kennedy Institute of
Rheumatology, London

CHAPMAN AND HALL
London

A HALSTED PRESS BOOK

JOHN WILEY & SONS
New York

First published in 1974
by Chapman and Hall Ltd
11 New Fetter Lane, London EC4P 4EE
© 1974 M.W. Steward
Typeset by E.W.C. Wilkins Ltd., London and
printed in Great Britain by William Clowes & Sons Ltd.,
London, Colchester and Beccles

Cop. 1

Library of Congress Cataloging in Publication Data

Steward, Michael W
 Immunochemistry.

 (Outline studies in biology)
 Bibliography: p
 1. Immunochemistry. I. Title. [DNLM: 1. Immunochemistry.
QW504 S849i 1974]
QR182.S73   574.2'9   74-4104
ISBN 0-470-82470-0

BST
Nat

Contents

1 Introduction

It has been known for a long time that contact with infectious organisms such as bacteria or viruses results in an individual becoming immune to subsequent re-infection with the same agent. Immunity to such infectious agents depends both upon the production of antibodies (γ globulins which react with the agent and assist in its elimination) *and* cell-mediated immune mechanisms. Whilst it is clear that these humoral and cellular aspects of immunity are interdependent it seems that modern research immunologists have segregated themselves into one or other of these fields. This dichotomy in immunology is not a new phenomenon. Indeed, it was not until the work of Wright (1903) showing that antibodies ('opsonins') actually aided the cell-mediated phagocytosis of bacteria described earlier by Metchnikoff (1883), that a compromise between the two hypotheses of immunity was achieved. However, whilst not aiming to condone or contribute to this segregation of research interests, the subject matter of this book is predominantly concerned with the humoral aspects of immunity; the cellular aspects will be dealt with in a further volume of this series.

The history of the study of antibodies goes back as far as 1890 when Von Behring first studied the neutralization of bacterial toxins by horse antitoxin antibodies. At about this time Paul Ehrlich, pioneer of immunochemistry became the first person to study quantitatively the precipitation reaction of toxin and antitoxin. It was his interest in immunological precipitation reactions which led the great physical chemist Arrhenius to be the first to use the word *immunochemistry*. In publishing in 1907 a series of lectures entitled 'Immunochemistry' he stated:

'I have given to these lectures the title 'Immunochemistry' and wish with this word to indicate that the chemical reactions of substances that are produced by the injection of foreign substances into the blood of animals, i.e. by immunisation, are under discussion in these pages. From this it follows also, that the substances with which these products react as proteins and ferments, are to be here considered with respect to their chemical properties.'

This definition is still applicable to modern immunochemistry and could be rephrased in modern terms as the study of the chemistry of antigens and antibodies and of the mechanism of their interaction.

Our concepts have of course, broadened from those of the early immunochemists who considered antibodies and antigens as homogeneous substances — even serum was considered as a single '*antigen*'. We now know that this is very far from the truth and that even simple purified antigens such as albumin have several antigenic determinants. The use of synthetic antigens of defined structure is helping to establish some of the molecular requirements for antigenicity. Antibodies are notoriously heterogeneous with regard to structure and function and it is this fact which has hindered the detailed study of the chemical structure and synthesis of immunoglobulins. The discovery of myeloma proteins — homogeneous proteins representing a single immunoglobulin species in patients with myelomatosis — has greatly aided the study of antibody structure. Even so the question of whether myeloma proteins are truly representative of antibody still remains unanswered. One of the aspects of the immune response which has challenged immunochemists is the nature of the genetic control of such a system which enables antibodies to be produced with specificity towards a constantly changing antigenic environment. Whether the ability to exhibit such variation is a result of somatic mutation of a limited number of genes transmitted in the germ line, or whether the germ line carries all the necessary genes for antibody diversity remains to be elucidated.

In spite of the enormous advances made in the field of immunochemistry within the last few years, particularly in our knowledge of the structure, synthesis and function of antibodies and in preliminary studies of the location, structure and composition of the antibody binding site, much remains to be established.

It is against this general background that this book is written. Its aim is to give the reader a general outline of the considerable amount of immunochemical knowledge available and to convey something of the direction which current research is taking.

2 Antigens

The term 'antigen' is commonly used in two ways. Firstly to describe a substance which, when injected into an appropriate animal, elicits the production of circulating antibodies or changes in cellular reactivity such as delayed hypersensitivity, and, secondly, to describe a substance which has the property of reacting with antibody i.e. antigenic specifity. It is clear that these two characteristics are not the same. Some substances have the capacity to react with antibodies but do not themselves elicit antibody formation and similarly there are substances which provoke an immune response in some animals (responders) but not in others (non-responders). Thus in order to describe a substance according to its ability to induce an immune response, the immune responsiveness of the host must be taken into consideration. The term 'immunogen' has recently been used to describe this aspect of the antigenicity of a substance. Thus, in a responder, an antigenic substance is immunogenic whereas in a non-responder, it is non-immunogenic. The term antigenicity therefore defines two properties of a substance: (i) immunogenicity and (ii) antigenic specificity. Certain areas on the antigen molecule termed antigenic determinants are responsible for these properties of immunogenicity and antigenic specificity. These determinants have a three dimensional structure with which the antibody binding site reacts and an antigen may have several such determinants which are not necessarily identical.

Bacteria and blood cells were the most commonly studied antigens during the pioneering days of immunology. Subsequently bacterial toxins and other soluble plant and animal products were investigated and at the same time some idea of the chemical nature of these natural antigens was being obtained. These were generally classified as proteins, lipoproteins, glycoproteins or polysaccharides. The more recent application of sophisticated chemical and biochemical techniques for the isolation, purification and synthesis of antigenic substances has resulted in major advances in our understanding of the nature of antigens.

Antigens may be considered [1,2] as belonging to one of three classes: A. *Natural* antigens, B. *Artificial* antigens and C. *Synthetic* antigens (See Table 2.1)

Table 2.1 Classes of antigens

Class of Antigen	Origin	Examples
Natural	Plants, Bacteria, Animals.	Particulate: blood cells, bacteria, viruses. Soluble: toxins toxoids, proteins, carbohydrates, glycoproteins liproproteins.
Artificial	Chemically modified natural antigens.	Iodinated proteins, Protein-hapten conjugates. e.g. AZO & DNP – proteins.
Synthetic	Chemically synthethised molecules.	Polypeptides, Polyaminoacids, Multichain aminoacid copolymers.

These three broad categories of antigens will now be considered in outline, with examination of examples of antigens in each.

2.1 Natural antigens

2.1.1 Blood cells, viruses and bacteria

As mentioned above, the use of complex particulate natural antigens such as blood cells, bacteria and viruses has played an important role in the development of our understanding of the immune response. Indeed, such antigens as sheep red blood cells are still regularly used particularly in studies of antibody formation at the cellular level where the haemolytic plaque forming cell assay system of Jerne [3] facilitates the detection of antibody forming cells *in vitro*. The immunochemistry of red blood cell antigens is still the subject of a great deal of research interest both at the theoretical and applied level. With regard to the latter the study of the D red cell antigen (the antigen commonly involved in the haemolytic disease of newborn children) and of the kinetics of its reaction with the corresponding antibody has made a considerable contribution to the control of this disease by passive transfer of anti-D antibody to D negative (i.e. rhesus negative) mothers suspected of being sensitized with D positive cells [4].

The Tobacco Mosaic Virus (T.M.V.) was the first virus to be identified and crystallised and has been used as a multivalent antigen. The first electron microscopic demonstration of the antibody:antigen interaction employed this antigen. This virus is of particular interest to immunochemists since it consists of an RNA core and 2 130 identical polypeptide units (158 amino acids per unit of known sequence) as its protein coat.

The use of bacteria and viruses as antigens is still of considerable interest particularly where the chemical structure of the cell wall is known. For example the immunodominant group in the haemolytic streptococci groups A and C are known in detail (Section 2.1.3), and these antigens are being used in studies into the nature of the genetic control of antibody production. [1, 2, 3]

2.1.2 Proteins

Proteins (Table 2.2) were the first substances shown to be antigenic, and are still widely used as antigens.

Table 2.2 Commonly studied protein antigens

Protein	Molecular weight (approx)
TMV Subunit protein	17 000
Myoglobin	17 000
Flagellin	40 000 (& polymeric form)
Ovalbumin	44 000
Diptheria toxoid	65 000
Serum albumin	69 000
Transferrin	90 000
Globulins	170 000
Keyhole limpet haemocyanin	$2\text{-}7 \times 10^6$

Proteins are highly complex molecules which are readily obtained in a highly purified state from plants, animals and micro-organisms. However, very little is known about the precise nature of their multiple antigenic determinants. In spite of such limitations, studies employing protein antigens have made major contributions to our understanding of the immune response.

Attempts have been made to delineate some of the antigenic determinants of several proteins by limited proteolysis. Such a procedure yielded a peptide fragment from human serum albumin of molecular weight approx. 7 000 which contains one of the antigenic determinants of the parent molecule [5, 6]. Lack of detailed knowledge of the structure of proteins has hindered further study of this problem. However, myoglobin, a protein, whose amino acid sequence and conformation is known in detail, has been used for studies on the nature of its antigenic determinants. This protein which, unfortunately is not a particularly good immunogen, has a minimum of four antigenic determinants. Immunochemical studies of the whole molecule and peptide fragments from it [7] have revealed that there are two types of antigenic determinants in the molecule (i) 'sequential': a determinant comprised of an amino acid sequence in a random coil form and (ii) 'conformational': a determinant whose nature depends upon steric conformation. These aspects will be discussed in more detail in Section 2.4.

Immunochemical studies of the protein antigen Flagellin — isolated from the flagella of *Salmonella* organisms have given some clues as to the nature and location of its antigenic determinants. Cleavage of the monomeric form (40 000 molecular weight) with cyanogen bromide (which breaks peptide bonds involving the amino acid methionine) yields four fragments, one of which contains all the antigenic determinants of the native molecule [8]. Further studies are needed to define more precisely the nature of these determinants. Similar studies have been carried out on the sub-unit protein of the Tobacco Mosaic Virus which has a molecular weight of approx. 17 000. The binding activity of peptide fragments of the unit protein with antibodies to the whole molecule have been studied in an attempt to localise the antigenically active site of the molecule.

In addition to the use of enzymically and chemically produced peptides for the study of the antigenic determinants on proteins, the technique of chemical modification has also been used. The effect of various chemical treatments on the antigenicity of the protein has been studied including denaturation, oxidation, reduction, digestion, deamination, esterification, acylation and halogenation [9]. Proteins treated in this way exhibit reduced reactivity with antibody to the native molecule, but interpretation of such results is a problem. The question of whether the effect is due to modification of a specific site or merely a conformational alteration as a result of the treatment is very difficult to answer.

It is clear that in spite of the wide use of proteins as antigens over many years, there is as yet very little information on the antigenic nature of these highly complex molecules and as such this field remains one of great challenge for immunochemists. Simple proteins and naturally occurring peptides have also been studies as antigens. These include insulin, glucagon, gastrin, calcitonin, bradykinin, angiotensin, vasopressin, adrenocorticotrophic hormone and growth hormone. In general, they are poor immunogens and require that their immunogenicity be enhanced in order to induce antibody formation either by immunization with adjuvants or by chemical coupling to natural or synthetic carrier molecules. Such poor immunogenicity has been ascribed to the low molecular weight of the peptides. The measurement of several of these substances in human serum by radioimmunoassay has useful clinical application. Their poor immunogenicity poses quite a problem since such assays require a potent (high affinity) antibody in order to be sufficiently sensitive.

2.1.3 Carbohydrates

Most types of bacteria have serologically active carbohydrates on or in their cell walls. Such carbohydrates react with antibody raised to the bacteria but are not themselves immunogenic i.e. they behave as haptens (See Section 2, 2). In other cases isolated carbohydrates such as the group A and group C carbohydrates of meningococci and the pneumococcal polysaccharides are immunogenic in man. Other carbohydrates such as dextrans, levans and teichoic acids have also been shown to be immunogenic in man. The molecular weight of the carbohydrate appears to be particularly important in the immunogenicity of these substances with repeating antigenic determinants. Dextrans — polymers of D-glucose, have been widely studied in this regard and it has been shown that dextrans of molecular weight less than 50 000 are far less immunogenic in man than those of molecular weight 90 000 or above [10]. The molecular weight of type III pneumococcal polysaccharide has to exceed 18 000 to induce an immune response in mice [11]. The group specific carbohydrates A and C from streptococcal cell walls have been extensively studied as antigens. The immunization of rabbits with vaccine prepared from heat-killed, pepsin digested Group A or Group C organisms elicits the formation of antibody to the group specific carbohydrate. The group A carbohydrate consists of repeating N-acetyl glucosamine-rhamnose units (17 moles of N-acetyl glucosamine and 38 modes rhamnose) and has a molecular weight of approximately 10 000. The N-acetylglucosamine is the immunodominant group. Group C carbohydrate has a similar structure consisting of N-acetylgalactosamine-rhamnose units with N-acetylgalactosamine as the immunodominant moiety. The exquisite specificity of the antibodies formed is illustrated by the fact that N-acetyl glucosamine inhibits the precipitation of A carbohydrate by antibody to A vaccine, whereas N-acetylgalactosamine does not. The converse is true with the C carbohydrate [12]. The group specific streptococcal and pneumococcal carbohydrates are particularly interesting to immunochemists because rabbit antibodies to such carbohydrates are, unlike normal antibodies, frequently of restricted molecular heterogeneity [11]. The study of such antibodies is making a major contribution to our knowledge of the genetic control of immunoglobulin structure and synthesis.

2.1.4 Lipids
The immunogenicity of a purified lipid has never been convincingly demonstrated and it appears that in order to obtain antibody to a lipid, it has to be complexed with larger macromolecular structures such as proteins, synthetic polypeptides or red blood cells.

2.1.5 Nucleic acids
Within the last two decades, nucleic acids have been of great interest to biochemists, and the finding of antibodies to nucleic acids in the serum of patients with the disease *systemic lupus erythematosus* (SLE) aroused the interest of immunochemists in these complex molecules. SLE is a disease with numerous immunological abnormalities including the presence of antinuclear and antinucleic acid antibodies in the serum. Immune complexes of anti DNA antibody and DNA are frequently deposited in the glomeruli of the kidneys. Antibodies to nucleic acid antigens have been sucessfully obtained experimentally only after conjugation to carriers such as methylated bovine serum albumin, proteins or synthetic polyamino-acids. In spite of considerable interest in the immunochemistry of these materials the precise nature of their immunogenic properties remains to be defined.

2.2 Artificial antigens
It will be clear from what has been said above that in order to gain knowledge of the chemical basis for immunogenicity, the problem of the enormous complexity of natural antigens has to be overcome. One approach which has been used by immunochemists to answer this problem is that of chemical modification of natural antigens to produce artificial antigens. Thus, the substitution of small determinant groups of known chemical structure on to protein antigens has provided much of our information on the nature of the specificity of immunological reactions.

It has been known since the early part of this century, that proteins lose their species specificity when heavily iodinated. Antibodies

Table 2.3 Examples of common haptens

Group	Structure	Mode of coupling to carrier
azobenzoate	$R - N = N -\langle\bigcirc\rangle - COO^-$	azo bonds with aromatic rings of tryosine, histidine, and $\epsilon\text{-}NH_2$ of lysine
azobenzenearsonate	$R - N = N -\langle\bigcirc\rangle - AsO_3H^-$	
azobenzensulphonate	$R - N = N -\langle\bigcirc\rangle - SO_3^-$	
dinitrophenol	$R -\langle\bigcirc\rangle\substack{NO_2 \\ NO_2}$	nucleophilic substitution using halogen derivative, i.e. 2, 4-dinitrofluoro-benzene
trinitrophenol	$R -\langle\bigcirc\rangle\substack{NO_2 \\ NO_2 \\ NO_2}$	NH_2 groups of lysine
4-hydroxy-3-iodo-5-nitrophenacetyl	$R - N = N - COCH_2 -\langle\bigcirc\rangle\substack{I \\ OH \\ NO_2}$	azide reacts with NH_2 groups of lysine

R = protein   R = protein

to such iodinated proteins are directed mainly to the iodinated tyrosine residues common to such iodinated proteins. However, it was not until the classical immunochemical experiments of Karl Landsteiner [13] using well defined small molecules coupled to proteins, that information regarding the specificity of immunological reactions began to accumulate. Landsteiner first introduced the term 'hapten' to describe 'specific protein free substances which, although reactive *in vitro*, induced no, or only slight antibody response. For serologically active substances of this sort, in contradistinction to the protein antigens, which possess both properties, the term *'hapten'* has been proposed'.

Although the term 'hapten' is frequently applied to low molecular weight aromatic substances (Table 2.3), the above definition indicates that the term can be applied to any substance which does not elicit antibody

formation by itself (i.e. is not immunogenic) but is capable of reacting with antibodies synthesised against a complete immunogenic molecule. Substances which are as varied as aromatic compounds, certain drugs (Penicillin), oligosaccharides, nucleic acids and nucleotides, peptides and lipids can all be haptens.

Although the role of conformation of configuration in immunogenicity will be discussed in more detail in section 2.4, the pioneering work of Landsteiner on the serological specificity of different azo-proteins will be mentioned briefly here. He demonstrated that when the three isomers of aminobenzene sulphonic acid (ortho, meta and para) were diazotized and coupled to protein (horse serum protein) and injected into rabbits, the antibodies so produced were able to differentiate between the three isomers. Thus antibodies to the horse protein containing the meta azobenzene sulphonate group gave a good precipitate with a different carrier protein bearing the meta isomer, but only poor precipitates with the two other isomers. In similar experiments, Landsteiner and Van der Scheer [14] were able to demonstrate by inhibition of precipitation, that the antibody to the sulphonic acid hapten could distinguish between the sulphonic acid hapten and an azobenzene hapten in which the sulphonate group was replaced by an arsonate or carboxylate group. These experiments further demonstrate the exquisite specificity of the antibody-antigen interaction.

The use of azocoupling to produce conjugates is not only applicable to aromatic amines but can be used to couple carbohydrate derivatives to proteins. Indeed, Landsteiner was able to demonstrate the serological specificity of D- and L-tartaric acids by synthesising the two isomeric diazo-tartranilic acids and coupling these to carrier protein. Antibodies to these conjugates could distinguish between these and the D- and L-isomers. Such work is an excellent example of the contribution that studies on artificial antigens have made to our knowledge of the specificity of the immunological response.

Before going on to discuss the use of completely synthetic antigens, the results of studies in which chemical groups were attached to the poor immunogen gelatin in order to investigate their effect on its immunogenicity will be briefly considered. The results of several studies are summarized in Table 2.4 and detailed references can be found in [15]. It is clear that the addition of a wide range of chemical groups can generally enhance the immunogenicity of gelatin. When the aromatic amino acid tyrosine is incorporated at a level of 2% into gelatin, the immunogenicity of gelatin itself is greatly enhanced. However, at levels of 10% tyrosine, the gelatin is again highly immunogenic but the specificity of the antibodies produced is directed towards

Table 2.4 The effect of coupling haptens and peptides on the immunogenicity of gelatin

Group coupled	Effect of immunogenicity
Sugar residues e.g. arabinose	–
cellulose-glycol	–
Sugar residues + tyrosine	↑
Aromatic compounds:- e.g. diazonium compounds	↑
benzoic acid	–
phenylisocyanate	–
Amino Acids:- D-tyrosine, L-tyrosine	↑
phenylalanine, methionine,	↑
tryptophan lysine, glutamine, alanine, serine	
Polyamino Acids:- polytyrosine, polyphenylalanine,	↑
polytryptophan, polyglycine polyalanine, polyglutamic acid, polylysine	–
Peptides:- leucine – glutamic acid, lysine-glutamic acid, tyrosine – glutamic acid	↑

↑ = increased immunogenicity
– = no effect on immunogenicity

tyrosyl peptides and not to gelatin [1]. Such studies, although providing some indication of the nature of immunogenicity, have obvious limitations. The introduction of techniques to produce completely synthetic antigens has led to a rapid advance in our understanding of the molecular basis of immunogenicity.

2.3 Synthetic antigens

From the preceding discussion it will be clear that studies into the precise chemical nature of what confers the immunogenic and antigenic properties to natural antigens such as proteins has been hampered by their extreme complexity. Valuable information on the specificity of the immune response has been obtained using artificial antigens but it was the availability of synthetic linear and branched polymers and copolymers of amino acids during the last 10—15 years, which has contributed greatly to our understanding of the molecular basis of immunogenicity. By studying the effects of precise changes in the chemical structure of these antigens, it has been possible to delineate many of the molecular characteristics which influence immunogenicity. Many such synthetic antigens have been tested in several species including mice, rabbits, guinea pigs, rats and humans and review articles should be consulted for detailed information. A summary of the types of synthetic antigens used in immunochemical studies is shown in Table 2.5.

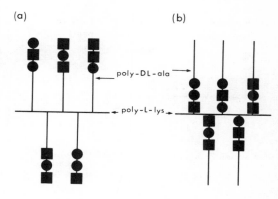

Fig. 2.1 Multichain copolymers of poly (tyr, glu)-poly-DL-ala-poly-L-lys. (a) immunogenic form (b) non-immunogenic form. (After [1]).

Table 2.5 Synthetic polypeptide antigens

Type	Example
Homopolymer	poly L-pro
Linear polypeptide	poly $glu^{56} lys^{38} tyr^6$
Random copolymer	$(pro^{66} gly^{34})$ n
Ordered sequence or periodic polymer (α helix)	(tyr-ala-glu) n
Multichain (branched) copolymer	poly (tyr-glu)-poly-DL-ala-poly-lys

An example of the structure of an immunogenic multichain (branched) copolymer poly (try-glu)-poly-DL-alanine-poly-L-lysine used by Sela [1] is shown in Figure 2.1(a). Here, tyrosine and glutamic acid residues are attached to the external part of the poly-DL-alanine-poly-L-lysine backbone (which by itself is not immunogenic). If the same amino acids are attached to the poly-L-lysine backbone directly and the poly-DL-alanine peptide then added (Fig. 2.1(b)) the resulting polypeptide is non-immunogenic. This illustrates the need for the immunologically important groups to be accessible in order to elicit antibody formation. Work from the

same author's laboratory has also shown that the same tripeptide (L-tyr-ala-L-glu) can be synthetically made either into a branched copolymer (an immunogen with sequential determinants) by attaching it to the side chains of poly-DL-ala-poly-L-lysine (Fig. 2.2(a)) or into an ordered sequence (or periodic polymer) which exists as an α-helix giving an immunogen with conformational determinants. (Fig. 2.2(b)). Antibodies to the sequential determinants do not cross react with the conformational determinants and vice versa, showing the importance of conformation in immunogenicity and antigenic specificity.

These examples serve to illustrate the type of studies which can be carried out with synthetic antigens. The kind of information obtained from such investigations on the molecular basis of immunogenicity and antigenic specificity will be summarized in the following section.

15

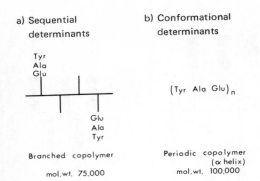

a) Sequential
determinants

Tyr
Ala
Glu

Glu
Ala
Tyr

Branched copolymer

mol. wt. 75,000

b) Conformational
determinants

$(Tyr \ Ala \ Glu)_n$

Periodic copolymer
(α helix)
mol. wt. 100,000

Fig. 2.2 Synthetic sequential and conformational antigenic determinants. (After [1]).

2.4 Molecular basis for immunogenicity and antigenic specificity

Sela has said [1]

'our knowledge of many molecular parameters — such as composition, size, shape, accessibility, electrical charge, optical configuration and steric conformation — controlling antigenicity, that is immunogenicity and antigenic specificity, has increased in recent years, and much of this advance is due to synthetic antigens. The relative simplicity of these molecules facilitates the interpretation of the results obtained with them, and sometimes permits the detection of effects such as genetic variations in immune response, which are not easily observable with complex natural antigens.'

In this section our present understanding of the role of the above parameters in controlling antigenicity will be briefly summarized.

2.4.1 Size

At one time it was thought that molecular weights below 5–10,000 were not immunogenic.

This is probably true for protein antigens but other molecules of molecular weight as low as 450 have been shown to be immunogenic (Table 2.6) either as evidenced by tests for antibody formation or alteration in cellular reactivity.

Table 2.6 Immunogens of low molecular weight

Immunogen	Molecular Weight	Species immunized
poly-Glu^{50}-Ala^{40}-Tyr^{10}	4 000	rabbit
tri-dinitrophenyl bacitracin	1 928	guinea pig
Angiotensin	1 031	guinea pig
p-azobenzenearsonate-tri-L-tyrosine	750	rabbit, guinea pig
p-azobenzenarsonate-N-acetyl-L-tyrosine	451	guinea pig

2.4.2 Composition

Homopolymers of α-amino acids are not generally immunogenic but polymers of two amino acids are immunogenic in rabbits and guinea pigs. Excellent immunogens have been obtained with polymers consisting of three or four amino acids. The coupling of tyrosine and phenylalanine to gelatin greatly increases its immunogenicity (Section 2.2). Similar effects are obtained using cyclohexylalanine (in which the aromatic rings of phenylalanine are replaced by cyclohexane rings) indicating that it is the ring structure rather than the aromaticity which makes tyrosine and phenylalanine immunogenically important. The presence of aromatic amino acids such as tyrosine in synthetic polypeptides, although generally increasing the amount of antibody produced, is not critical for their immunogenicity.

2.4.3 Steric conformation

It has been recognised for a long time that the spatial arrangement of proteins is important in antigenic specificity since denatured proteins react poorly, if at all, with antibodies directed to the native molecules. Work with synthetic polypeptides (see Fig. 2.2) clearly demonstrates that the immune system is capable of distinguishing between a sequential or random coil determinant and a conformational determinant (e.g. as an α-helix) even though the same amino acids are involved (the tripeptide tyr-ala-glu). Although there is no cross precipitation between the two systems, circular dichroism studies have shown [16] that when antibodies to the α-helical structure react with the random coil polypeptide, a conformational change may occur inducing a helical tendency in the random coil, and this has been termed transconformation. Similar antibody induced conformational changes in cross reacting antigens have been demonstrated with the antiapomyoglobin-myoglobin system. This reaction results in the release of ferrihaem from myoglobin as a result of conformational changes induced by the antibody [17].

Antibodies to the nonapeptide bradykinin, raised in rabbits by immunization with a branched chain copolymer of the peptide and poly-L-lysine, have been used to study the role of conformation in antigenic specificity [18]. The ability of various bradykinin analogues to bind with these antibodies was determined. Analogues in which changes in the amino acid side chains resulted in alteration of conformation (i.e. at proline or glycine residues) greatly altered the ability to bind to the antibody whereas substitutions resulting in charge or hydrophobicity changes did not effect the binding. Other evidence on the role of conformation in determining specificity is available, for example the elegant work of Arnon and Sela [19] on antibodies to the 'loop peptide' of hen egg white lysozyme (Fig. 2.3).

The isolated peptide containing the sequence 64-83 of lysozyme has been called the 'loop' peptide since it has the disulphide bridge between residues 64-80. When conjugated to multi poly-DL-ala-poly-lysine the

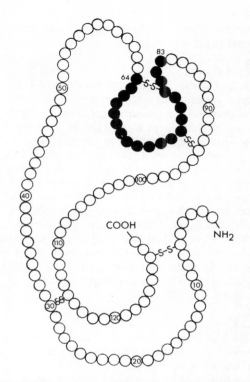

Fig. 2.3. The amino acid sequence of hen egg-white lysozyme showing the loop peptide (●—●). (Redrawn from (1)).

resulting conjugate elicited antibodies to native lysozyme in rabbits and goats. Antibodies of similar specificity could be isolated from serum of animals immunized with lysozyme using a preparation of insolubilized 'loop' peptide ('loop' peptide coupled to bromacetyl cellulose). These isolated antibodies still reacted with lysozyme and this reaction could be inhibited by the 'loop' peptide but *not* by the open chain peptide derived from the 'loop' by reduction and carboxymethylation. This indicates that the antibodies to the 'loop' are recognizing a specific steric conformation rather than just an amino-acid sequence. These workers have shown similar results with antibodies raised to a completely

17

synthetic 'loop' peptide of virtually identical amino acid sequence [20].

2.4.4 Charge
Several studies in which the net charge of synthetic antigens was systematically varied by alterations in amino acid composition have revealed that charge is not a requirement for immunogenicity and that in general, charge does not affect amounts of antibody produced. However, highly charged molecules are weakly immunogenic. It is interesting to note that there is an inverse relationship between the net electric charge of immunogenic molecules and the charge of the antibodies produced to them. Thus antibodies to basic *p*- azobenzenearsonate conjugates induced the production of relatively acidic antibodies whereas acidic p-azobenzene arsonate conjugates elicited more basic antibodies.

2.4.5 Optical configuration
The high degree of stereospecificity of antibodies in their reaction with antigen has been discussed in Section 2.3. The role of optical configuration in immunogenicity has been studied using synthetic polypeptide antigens. Polymers of D-amino acids are less immunogenic than those made up of the corresponding L-isomers. The attachment of L-amino acid residues to the outside of a synthetic macromolecule consisting of D-amino acids converts it into a good immunogen. Conversely, a macromolecule consisting of predominantly L-amino acids but having side chains terminating in D-amino acids is a very poor immunogen [21]. It seems that the poor immunogenicity of the D-amino acid polymers is due to their incomplete catabolism and retention in the animal for long periods of time. Slow release subsequently results in immune unresponsiveness.

2.4.6 Physical form
The physical form of an antigen when injected into an animal is of great importance in determining whether or not it will be immunogenic. Proteins, nucleic acids and synthetic antigens have different immunogenicity when in the aggregated or unaggregated form. Bovine γ globulin in the aggregated form is a good immunogen in mice but ultracentrifuged material, which is aggregate-free, induces unresponsiveness. Many antigens which are not immunogenic when administered in physiologic saline are highly immunogenic when incorporated in Freund's adjuvant (a water in oil emulsion in which killed, dried *Mycobacterium tuberculosis* are suspended) or adsorbed on to alum precipitates.

2.5 The size of the antigenic determinant
The approximate size of the region of an antigen which is in actual combination with the antibody binding site has been estimated by several workers using different antigens. In general the method of estimating the determinant size has been to inhibit the binding of antibody to homologous antigen using inhibitors of increasing size. For example, the size of the determinant in the human dextran-antidextran system has been shown to be equivalent to six glucopyranose rings by inhibition studies using an ordered series of oligosaccharides. Data from various systems shows that the size of the determinant in each is remarkably similar.

2.6 Cellular considerations
In addition to the molecular aspects which affect immunogenicity (Section 2.4), the immunological state of the host must be considered. It is now very clear that in the animal which is genetically capable of responding to an antigen the production of an immune response involves three types of cells which cooperate in the production of antibody: (1) thymus-derived (T) lymphocytes, (2) bone-marrow-derived (B)

Table 2.7 Approximate size of the determinants of various antigen

Antigen	Composition & approximate size of determinant Å	
Dextran	6 sugar residues	34 × 12 × 7
Nucleic Acid	4-5 purine or pyrimidine residues	15 × 20
Bacillus anthracis	hexapeptide	36 × 10 × 6
poly-ala-BSA	pentalanine	25 × 11 × 6.5
Poly-lys-RSA	penta(hexa)lysine	27 × 72 × 6.5
Poly-lys-phosphoryl-BSA	pentalysine	27 × 17 × 6.5

lymphocytes, and (3) macrophages (see section 3.4.1). During this response there is a phase in which antigen is recognized via receptors on lymphoid cells which are capable of specifically binding the antigen.

These cooperation and recognition reactions differ according to the nature of the antigen. T-lymphocytes have a function as 'helper cells' in the immune response where they are involved in the triggering of B-cells by antigen. Not all antigens require such T-cell helper effects and examples of 'thymus-independent' antigens are the lipopolysaccharide of gram-negative bacteria, pneumococcal polysaccharide and the synthetic antigen polyvinyl pyrrolidone. These antigens have the property of repeating antigenic determinants. Natural antigens such as immuno-globulin, albumin, and erythocytes generally require helper effects and are termed 'thymus-dependent' antigens.

The presentation of the antigen in an aggregate-free form or in very high doses may result in an animal being made unresponsive (tolerant) to an antigen to which it normally produces antibody. It appears that thymus cells can be made unresponsive more easily than bone marrow cells, and that the duration of such unresponsiveness is far longer in the thymus cells [23]. The mechanisms by which cells are triggered to produce antibody or to become unresponsive are unknown.

References

1. Sela, M. (1969), *Science* **166**, 1365.
2. Sela M. (1966), *Advanc. Immunol.* **5**, 29.
3. Jerne, N.K., & Nordin, A.A. (1963), *Science* **140**, 405.
4. Hughes Jones, N.C. (1967), *Immunology*, **12**, 565.
5. Press, E. and Porter R.F. (1962) *Biochem. J.* **83**, 172.
6. Lapresle & Webb (1965), *Biochem. J.* **95**, 245 and Lapresle & Goldstein (1969) *J. Immunol.* **102**, 733.
7. Crumpton, M.J. (1967), in 'Antibodies to Biologically active Molecules', (ed. B. Cinader), vol. 1. p. 61, Pergamon Press, New York.
8. Parish, C.R., Wostar, R. Jnr., & Ada, B.L. (1969), *Biochem. J.*, **113**, 501
9. Boyd, W.C. (1966), *Fundamentals of Immunology* p. 135–141, Wiley-Interscience, New York.
10. Kabat, E.A. & Bezer, A.E. (1958) *Arch. Biochem. Biophys.* **78**, 306.
11. McMaster, P.R.B., Schade, A.L., Finnerley, J.F., Caldwell, M.B. & Prescott, B. (1970), *Fed. Proc.* **29**, 812.
12. Krause, R.M. (1970), *Advance. Immunol.* **12**, p. 3.
13. Landsteiner, K. (1945), *The Specificity of Serological Reactions.* Havard Univ. Press. Cambridge, Mass.
14. Landsteiner, K. & van der Scheer, J. (1936), *J. exp. Med.* **63**, 325.
15. Gill, T.J. III, (1972), in *Immunogenicity, (Physicochemical & biological aspects)* (F. Borek, Ed.) p. 5. North Holland, Amsterdam.
16. Schechter, B., Conway-Jacobs, A. & Sela, M. (1971). *European J. Biochem.* **20**, 321.
17. Crumpton, M.J. (1965), *Biochem. J.* **100**, 223.
18. Spragg, J., Schroder, E. Stewart, M.J., Austen, K.F. & Haleer, E. (1967), *Biochemistry* **6**, 3933.
19. Arnon, R. & Sela, M. (1969), *Proc. Nat. Acad. Sci.* (USA) **62**, 163.
20. Arnon, R., Maron, E., Sela, M. & Anfinsen, C.B. (1971), *Proc. Nat. Acad. Sci.* (USA) **68**, 1950.

21. Jaton, J.L. & Sela, M. (1968), *J. Biol. Chem.* **243**, 5616.
22. Kabat, E.A. (1966), *J. Immunol.* **97**, 1.
23. Weigle, W.O. (1973) *Advanc. Immunol.* **16**, 61.

3 Immunoglobulins and antibodies

Although the work of Von Behring and co-workers (1890) had demonstrated the presence of antitoxin (or antibody) in the serum of immunized animals, it was not until 1938 that significant advances in the knowledge of the chemical nature of antibodies were made. At this time, Tiselius and Kabat [1] demonstrated that the antibody activity of serum is associated with the γ-globulin fraction using the technique of electrophoresis developed by Tiselius in 1937. Subsequently it has been shown that antibodies are a heterogeneous group of proteins which can be subdivided into classes on the basis of differences in their structure. In the human, five classes of proteins with antibody activity, termed immunoglobulins, are recognized: immunoglobulin G (IgG), IgM, IgA, IgD and IgE. Similar classes of antibody exist in other species. The heterogenity of the immunoglobulins in normal serum has made structural studies very difficult. However, the occurrence of homogeneous immunoglobulins (considered to be structurally similar to normal antibodies) in the blood and urine of patients with myelomatosis and macroglobulinaemia has provided a unique source of large amounts of material for the study of immunoglobulin structure.

3.1 Isolation and purification of immunoglobulins and specific antibodies

In order to carry out chemical and physico-chemical studies on immunoglobulins and antibodies, adequate amounts of these materials have to be isolated and purified. This section will deal briefly with methods employed for such isolation. More detailed information can be obtained from references 1 and 2.

The immunoglobulins are plasma proteins which are highly heterogeneous with regard to structure, size, charge and biological activity. This has made their isolation and purification a challenging problem for immunochemists. Methods developed for the isolation of immunoglobulins from other plasma proteins and from each other make use of their basic nature, differing solubilities in various solvents and their relatively high isoelectric points (IgG: pI $= 5{\cdot}8 - 7{\cdot}3$). Examples of the protein separation techniques which have been applied to the isolation of immunoglobulins are shown in Table 3.1.

The use of any one of these techniques by itself will not yield a pure preparation of immunoglobulin and in general a combination of techniques is used. Fractional precipitation techniques using ammonium or sodium sulphate are commonly used to effect a concentration of crude immunoglobulins from serum. At certain concentrations of these neutral salts (for example $1{\cdot}2 - 1{\cdot}8$ molar for $(NH_4)_2SO_4$) proteins such as albumin remain in solution. Further purification of the immunoglobulin can be achieved using other techniques such as ion exchange chromatography, gel filtration, electrophoresis or gradient ultracentrifugation.

Table 3.1 Methods for immunoglobulin isolation

Method	Examples
A. Fractional precipitation	
(i) Neutral salts	Ammonium sulphate sodium sulphate
(ii) Organic solvents	Ethanol
(iii) Metal ions	Zinc
(iv) Organic cations	Rivanol (2-ethoxy-6, 9, diamino-acridine lactate)
B. Electrophoretic separation	
(i) Carrier free media	Free boundary electrophoresis
(ii) Solid support	Zone electrophoresis on cellulose, acrylamide, starch gel, Pevikon
C. Ion exchange chromatography	Diethylaminoethyl-cellulose Carboxymethyl cellulose
D. Gel Filtration	Sephadex G200
E. Ultracentrifugation	Preparative ultra-centrifugation on sucrose or salt gradients.

Initial separation of crude immunoglobulins may also be obtained by zone electrophoresis.

The purified immunoglobulins obtained in these ways are very heterogeneous with regard to their antibody specificities. For the isolation of specific antibody, the inclusion of a preparative step which utilizes the specificity of the reaction of antibody with its corresponding antigen is necessary. Two general methods are commonly employed. The first involves the preparation of specific immune precipitates of antibody and antigen, with subsequent dissociation of the antibody: antigen complex and separation of antigen and antibody. The second involves the use of an immunoadsorbent consisting of antigen which has been coupled to an insoluble matrix such as cellulose, sepharose or agarose. Antibody reacts with the insolubilized antigen and, after removal of unreacted protein by washing, the antibody is dissociated from the matrix. The reagents commonly used to dissociate antibody antigen bonds are glycine-HCl buffer pH2 and chaotrophic agents such as high concentrations of sodium chloride, iodide and thiocyanate. Care has to be taken not to denature the antibody during the dissociation procedure. Recently, techniques for the isolation of anti-hapten antibodies have been described where the antigen is trapped in a matrix of highly cross-linked polyacrylamide. Antibody diffuses through the polyacrylamide and reacts with the trapped antigen. After washing out unreacted material, the antibody is dissociated from the antigen by elution with low pH buffer.

Immunoglobulins and specific antibodies isolated in these ways have been used to produce the information described in this chapter and Chapter 4.

3.2 Detection and measurement of immunoglobulins and antibodies

There are many tests available for the detection and measurement of immunoglobulins and antibodies. In general such tests make use of the fact that after combination with antigen, antibodies will agglutinate red cells or particles coated with antigen or potentiate measureable biological reactions; or form precipitates which can be visualized in solution or gel. Some of these methods are shown in Table 3.2, together with the minimum amount of antibody which they can detect.

There is a wide variation in sensitivity of such tests depending upon which particular property of the antibody is being exploited (i.e. precipitation, agglutination etc.) The reaction of an antibody (Ab) with an antigen or antigenic determinant (Ag) to produce a complex (Ab Ag) can be represented as follows:-

$$Ab + Ag \underset{kd}{\overset{ka}{\rightleftharpoons}} AbAg$$

Table 3.2 Sensitivity of antibody detection methods (See [4] for references)

Method	Minimum amount antibody detectable (μg/ml.)
Precipitation:	
(i) ring test	20–30
(ii) optimal proportions	50
(iii) P-80 radioprecipitation	1·0
Gel diffusion:	
(i) double diffusion tube	20–50
(ii) single diffusion tube	12–110
(iii) double diffusion plate	40
(iv) single diffusion plate	10
Immunoelectrophoresis	100
Radioimmunoelectrophoresis	0·02
Crossed electrophoresis	100
Agglutination	0·1 – 120
Passive haemagglutination	0·03
Complement Fixation	0·1 – 1–0 μg
Passive cutaneous anaphylaxis	0·02
Farr binding [$(NH_4)_2 SO_4$ precipitation]	0·05 – 1·0
Antiglobulin precipitation	μg-ng/ml range
Immunoadsorbent	20
Radioimmunoassay	μg-ng/ml range

where *ka* is the association constant, *kd* the dissociation constant. This is the primary antibody-antigen reaction and several methods are available to detect and quantitate this interaction. After one of these primary interactions have occurred other secondary or tertiary manifestations [5] may or may not occur depending on the nature of the antibody being tested. Examples of secondary manifestations are precipitate formation, agglutination and complement fixation. Tertiary manifestations such as anaphylaxis or immune elimination of antigen are very far removed from the primary reaction and are greatly affected, for example, by host variations. Since many variables control both secondary and tertiary manifestations of the primary antibody antigen reaction, negative results with these tests occur even in the presence of antibody demonstrable by the primary tests. Therefore, since the results of primary binding tests are the only reliable guide to the presence or absence of antibody experiments requiring accurate estimations of antibody levels should include at least one such test [6]. Methods of antibody detection and quantitation are classified into primary, secondary and tertiary categories in Table 3.3.

Table 3.3 Classification of antibody detection methods (after [5])

Category	Method
Primary	Radioimmunoelectrophoresis. Farr binding. Antiglobulin technique. Fluorescence quenching, enhancement, polarization. Equilibrium dialysis.
Secondary	Gel diffusion. 'P-80' radioprecipitation. Agglutination. Complement fixation.
Tertiary	Passive cutaneous anaphylaxis. Arthus reaction. Immune elimination.

3.3 Immunoglobulin structure

Three groups of antibodies can be detected in serum by ultracentrifugation (a) proteins of molecular weight approximately 150 000 and a sedimentation coefficient of 7S (b) proteins of molecular weight approx. 300 0.00 (9–11S) and (c) 19S proteins of molecular weight approx 900 000. The 7S is the major group and consists predominantly of IgG. This immunoglobulin accounts for about 70% of the total serum immunoglobulins.

3.3.1. The basic four chain model for IgG

The first attempts to investigate the structure of antibodies were made by R.R. Porter (7) who demonstrated that when 7S rabbit antibodies were incubated with the proteolytic enzyme papain in the presence of cysteine three major fragments I, II and III were obtained. Using carboxymethylcellulose ion exchange chromatography to separate the fragments, Porter showed that one of these (fragment III) could be crystallized (subsequently called Fc 'fragment crystallizable') and that fragments I and II were identical to each other and unlike the Fc, were able to combine with the antigen. These observations thus accounted for the known valency of 2 for IgG antibodies and these fragments were subsequently termed Fab (fragment antigen binding). Nisonoff and his co-workers [8] showed that on treatment of 7S antibody with pepsin a bivalent 5S antibody fragment is produced which, when reduced yields two monovalent 3·5S fragments. Further studies by Porter and by G.M. Edelman showed that the constituent chains of immunoglobulin can be isolated by reduction of the interchain disulphide bonds with sulphydryl reagents in urea solution or by reduction followed by alkylation of the free SH groups and subsequent dissociation of non-covalent bonds by gel filtration in acid. These observations formed the basis on which Porter [9] postulated a four polypeptide chain structure for IgG (Figure 3.1).

Thus IgG consists of two heavy and two light chains linked by covalent disulphide bonds and other non-covalent forces (e.g. hydrogen bonding). The heavy chains of human IgG with 450 amino acid residues (M.Wt. 50 000) are approximately twice the size of the light chains which have 220 amino acid residues (M.Wt. 23 000). This general structure for IgG has been confirmed by electron microscopy of antibody to DNP complexed to bis-N-DNP-octamethylene diamine which is a bifunctional hapten molecule consisting of an eight-carbon chain with a dinitrophenol group at each end. In the presence of this reagent, anti-DNP

antibodies appear as three molecules linked by the (invisible) reagent via their Fab regions with the Fc parts of the molecule forming projections at the corner of the triangle thus formed. (Fig. 3.2.)

Digestion with pepsin removes the Fc from the corner of the structure. It was concluded from these studies that IgG is a flexible Y-shaped molecule made up of three rigid rods representing the Fab and Fc fragments [11]. The fragmentation of antibody by enzyme and chemical treatment is illustrated in Fig. 3.3.

It has been shown that this four chain structure is basic for all immunoglobulin classes and that although the light chains are similar in each case, the heavy chains are specific for each class. Thus γ heavy chains are specific for IgG, α for IgA, μ for IgM, δ for IgD and ε for IgE.

Light chains have been serologically separated into kappa (κ) and lambda (λ) types. It has been shown that in the human, 65% of immuno-globulins have κ light chains the remainder having the λ type. In any one immunoglobulin molecule the two light chains are always of the same type and both κ and λ types can be associated with any heavy chain class. It should be mentioned that the κ : λ ratio varies from species to species.

3.3.2 Immunoglobulin classes
The physicochemical properties of the human immunoglobulins are shown in Table 3.2 and the biological activities of the major immuno-globulin classes are discussed in Chapter 4.

It is clear that the immunoglobulins are physicochemically heterogeneous particularly with regard to molecular weight. This is in part due to the presence of polymeric forms (IgA and IgM) and also to differences in heavy chain structure. The structure of the major classes will be briefly discussed:

Immunoglobulin G IgG is quantitatively the most important serum immunoglobulin and

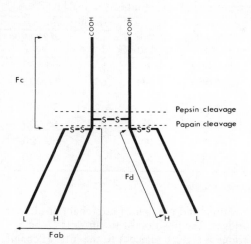

Fig. 3.1 Diagram of the fourchain structure for rabbit IgG suggested by R.R. Porter.

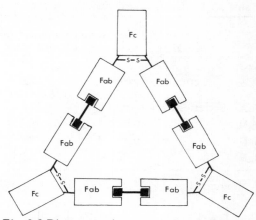

Fig. 3.2 Diagrammatic representation of anti-DNP antibody-antigen complex as seen in the electron microscope, showing the Y-shaped structure of the antibody (after [10]).

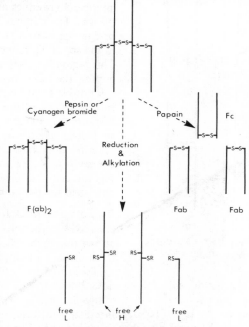

Fig. 3.3 Preparation of fragments of IgG by enzymic and chemical degradation.

Table 3.2 Physicochemical characteristics of human immunoglobulins (data from [12])

Class	Number of subclases	Mean Serum conc. mg/ml	Sedimentation coefficient	Molecular weight	Carbo-hydrate %	Heavy chain Type	Molecular weight
IgG	2	13·2	7S	160 000	2·9	γ	53 000
IgA	Serum 2	1·6	7S (9S, 11S, 13S)	170 000*	9·9	α1	56 000
IgA	Secretions 2	—	11S	390 000**	11·7	α2	52 000
IgM	2	0·9	19S	900 000	11·8	μ	65 000
IgD	2	0·1	7S	184 000	13·0	δ	69 700
IgE		0·00033	8S	188 000	11·6	ε	72 500

* Monomer IgA   ** 7S dimer plus secretory component

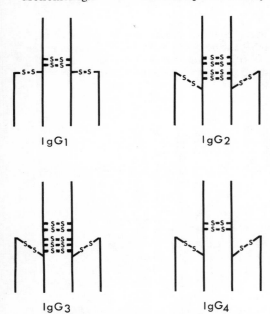

IgG1   IgG2

IgG3   IgG4

Fig. 3.4 Arrangement of interchain disulphide bridges in the four human IgG subclasses (after [13]).

has four known antigenically distinct subclasses of which IgGl is the major subclass (70% of the total IgG) followed by IgG2 (16%), IgG3 (10%) and IgG4 (4%). As shown in Fig. 3.4 there are marked differences in the

positions and number of interchain disulphide bridges. The position of the inter H-L chain bridge is almost adjacent to the inter H chain bridges in IgGl but in the other classes, the inter H-L chain bridge is of the order of 90 amino acid residues away from the inter H chain bridges. The number of inter H chain disulphide bridges varies from 2 to 5. These are clustered in the so-called 'hinge region' of the molecule. This region is rich in the amino acid proline (which confers the flexibility to the region) and is susceptible to proteolysis. The human IgG subclasses also differ in the antigens or genetic markers they express in their Fc regions. The subject of genetic markers will be discussed later in this chapter. At the present time subclasses of IgG are known in the mouse, guinea pig, rat, cow and sheep but have not been described for the rabbit.

Immunoglobulin A Immunoglobulins of the IgA class exist in the serum as the 7S monomer and also as polymeric 9S, 11S and 23S forms. IgA has a higher carbohydrate content than does IgG.

Two subclasses of human IgA have been described — IgA1 and IgA2 — on the basis of antigenic differences in the α chain. Another interesting difference is the absence of the H-L disulphide bond and the presence of L-L disulphide linked dimers in the IgA2 proteins bearing the Am + genetic marker or allotype [14](Fig. 3.5).IgA1 is the predominant subclass (80%) in serum. However, in secretions the

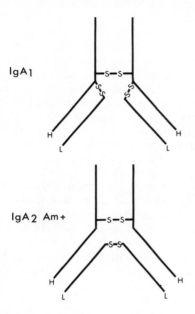

IgA₁

IgA₂ Am+

Fig. 3.5 Human IgA subclasses.

subclasses occur in approximately equal concentrations.

IgA exists in human secretions such as saliva, tears, intestinal secretions and colostrum where it is the major immuno-globulin. It is locally produced in the epithelial cells of the mucosae and exocrine glands. Secretory IgA is an 11S molecule of M.Wt. 385 000 which consists of two 7S IgA monomers plus an antigenically distinct component termed the 'secretory component'. Secretory component, a glyco-protein of M.Wt. 58 000, occurs in external secretions in both the free form and in association with the dimeric IgA. The mode of linkage of the secretory component to the two IgA subunits has yet to be

unravelled. However, it is thought that in human secretory IgA, both covalent and non-covalent binding to the Fc region of the IgA subunits involved. The function of this component is not known but some evidence suggests that it may confer resistance to proteolysis to the molecule [15]. It may also facilitate transport of the IgA across membranes into the secretions. The two monomeric constituents of human secretory IgA have been shown to have identical light chain types (κ or λ) even though the serum IgA molecules had either κ or λ [16]. This, together with other evidence, indicates that the secretory IgA is not randomly assembled from monomeric plasma IgA.

It is interesting to note that a protein called 'J (junction) chain' of molecular weight approxi-mately 25 000 has been described [17]. It con-sists of a single amino acid chain with a high cysteine (12 residues) and aspartic acid content and is considered to be involved in the formation of polymeric IgA and IgM. The precise way in which J chain is involved in poly-merisation has yet to be defined.

Immunoglobulin M IgM is a macroglobulin of molecular weight around 900 000 with a some-what faster electrophoretic mobility than the lower molecular weight globulins. Early studies on IgM had shown that reduction and alkylation of the molecule yielded stable subunits. Sub-sequent studies using carefully defined conditions of disulphide bond reduction have shown that the IgM molecule consists of five 7S subunits which are linked by intersubunit disulphide bonds. In addition to physicochemical infor-mation, the results of electron microscopic studies of IgM proteins from various species have led to the now widely accepted circular pentameric structure for IgM as shown in Figure 3.6.

J chain is thought to be involved in the formation of this polymeric molecule but the mechanism of this is unknown.

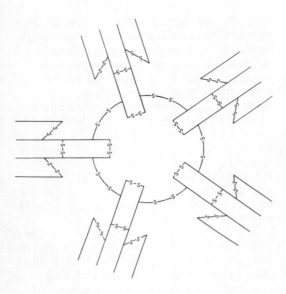

Fig. 3.6 Schematic representation of pentameric human IgM.

Immunoglobulins D and E Both IgD and particularly IgE occur in low levels in the serum, and this has made structural studies difficult. In addition, IgD is readily digested by the enzyme plasmin which has complicated the isolation of this immunoglobulin. However, the availability of myeloma proteins of both classes has now made structural studies possible and these immunoglobulins have the basic four-chain structure common to all immunoglobulins. They have higher molecular weights than IgG and IgA due, in part, to their larger heavy chains (see Table 3.2). In common with IgA and IgM, their carbohydrate content is significantly higher than that of IgG.

3.3.3 Amino acid sequence studies

The availability of homogeneous immunoglobulins from sera of patients with myelomatosis has enabled structural studies at the amino acid sequence level to be carried out. After IgG was shown to consist of light and heavy polypeptide chains which could be easily separated, it was demonstrated that the Bence-Jones protein found in the urine of many patients with myelomatosis were very similar to the light chains of the patient's myeloma IgG. Several of these proteins have been isolated and their amino acid sequences determined. Comparison of the results obtained from these proteins have shown that the L-chains can be divided into two regions — the V or variable region extending from amino acid positions 1-107 where there is a wide variability in amino acid sequence — and the C or constant region extending from position 108–214 where the sequences are remarkably similar. Characteristic sequence patterns in certain parts of the variable regions of light chains can be identified as belonging to the serologically defined κ or λ types. These regions are known as V_κ or V_λ respectively. A schematic representation of the constant and variable regions of human κ-Bence Jones proteins is shown in Fig. 3.7.

Closed circles represent positions where different amino acids have been found in other κ-Bence Jones proteins and open circles represent amino acid which are constant. There is less sequence data on heavy chains but these also have constant and variable regions. The constant region accounts for approximately 75% of the chain and the variable region the remainder. Edelman *et al* [19] in their determination of the complete amino acid sequence of a human IgG immunoglobulin showed that the variable region of the heavy chain extends from the N-terminus to approximately residue 120 and the constant region from residue 121 to 450. These workers noted that there were three regions within the constant region of the heavy chain which were very similar to each other and to the constant region of the light chains C_L. It has been suggested that these homology regions — C_H1, C_H2 and C_H3 of the

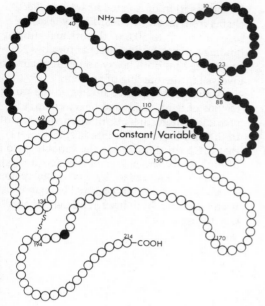

Fig. 3.7 Constant and variable regions of human κ light chains (after [18]).

heavy chain, and C_L of the light chain and the variable regions of H and L chains could each be folded into a compact 'domain' [20]. Each of these domains is stabilized by an intrachain disulphide bond and, it is proposed, has one or more functions e.g. antigen binding for the V_L and V_H domains; complement binding sites located in the C_H2 domain and macrophage binding for the C_H3 domain. A function for the C_H1 domain has yet to be precisely defined. Figure 3.8 shows an outline of the overall structure of the IgG protein sequenced by Edelman *et al* (1969) showing the variable and constant regions of both chains, homology regions, the disulphide bond arrangement and the position of carbohydrate. The domain

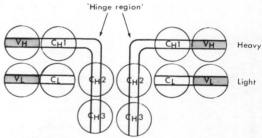

Fig. 3.9 The domain hypothesis (after [21]).

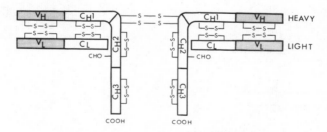

Fig. 3.8 Schematic representation of the general structure of human IgG_1 myeloma protein Eu. (after [19]).

29

hypothesis is represented diagrammatically in Figure 3.9. _frag antigen binding_

3.3.4 The antibody binding site

Since Porter demonstrated the antibody binding activity in the Fab fragments of immunoglobulins, a great deal of interest has been shown in the location and structure of the binding site.

Experiments to determine the ability of isolated chains of antibody to bind antigen have generally revealed that isolated heavy chains retain some activity and light chains little or none. However, using the sensitive technique of fluorescence enhancement (see section 4.3.3) antigen binding by L-chains has been demonstrated (See Fig. 3.10)

Recombination of isolated heavy and light chains from an anti-DNP antibody leads to recovery of up to 50% of the original antigen binding activity of the whole antibody [23] suggesting that both heavy and light chains are involved in the binding of antigen.

Amino acid sequence studies on the variable regions of light chains and heavy chains are providing interesting information with regard to the binding site of antibodies. It appears that there are areas within the variable regions of both heavy and light chains which are highly variable — the so called 'hypervariable' regions — two or three such hypervariable regions have been located in both heavy and light chains (see Figure 3.11.)

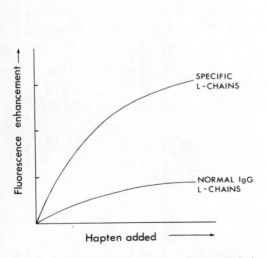

Fig. 3.10 Specific binding of analinonaphthalene sulphonate hapten by L-chains from anti-azonaphthalene sulphonate antibody (after [22]).

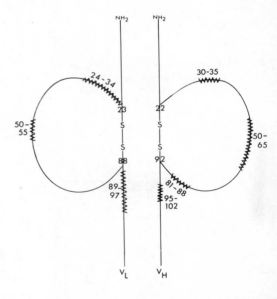

Fig. 3.11 The hypervariable regions of heavy and light chains. Numbers refer to amino acid residues (after [24]).

It is suggested that contact with antigen occurs at such regions and that the binding site is formed by the interaction of both chains. One experimental approach which is currently being actively used to provide support for this hypothesis and to obtain further information on the nature of the binding site is the technique of affinity labelling [25]. Essentially this involves reaction of antihapten antibody with a radioactive, chemically modified hapten which, by virtue of an additional reactive group, is able to form covalent bonds with amino acids in or near the antibody binding site. There are three major groups of affinity labelling reagents; (1), diazonium reagents, e.g. p-phenylarsonic acid diazonium fluoborate; (2), bromacetyl derivatives, e.g. α, N-bromoacetyl ε-N-DNP-L-lysine (BADL); and (3), arylnitrene reagents such as the 4azido-2-nitrophenyl (NAP) group. The principle of the method is shown in Figure 3.12.

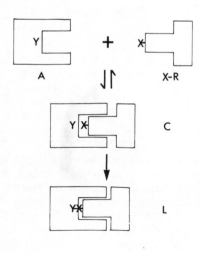

Fig. 3.12 Principle of affinity labelling (after [25]).

The affinity label (X–R) first forms a reversible complex C with the antibody binding site A. Whilst in the site, it forms a covalent bond with a suitable amino acid residue Y forming the stable complex L (i.e. $A + X - R \rightleftharpoons C \rightarrow L$). Subsequent digestion and analysis of the molecule allows the labelled amino acid to be characterized. By such methods early results showed that the tyrosine residues in the variable regions of both heavy and light chains are labelled, with the ratio of labelling of heavy: light ranging from 1 : 3 to 1 : 4. Several affinity labelling reagents are now being actively used, and results seem to indicate that the hypervariable regions are indeed susceptible to labelling. Studies of this type should help to define the amino acids involved in the binding site. Homogeneous antibodies of defined specificity also provide another approach to the study of the binding site [26]. However, the precise determination of the three-dimensional structure of the antibody site requires the additional use of X-ray crystallographic techniques.

3.3.5 Allotypes and idiotypes
From what has been discussed so far, it will be evident that the structure of immunoglobulins poses the intriguing question as to the nature of the genetic control of their synthesis and the origin of antibody variability. Before discussing this aspect of immunochemistry, consideration must be given to allotypes and idiotypes, both of which have made and are making significant contributions to the study of the genetic control of immunoglobulin synthesis

Allotypes Allotypes were first described in 1956 by Oudin [27] in rabbit immunoglobulins and in the same year Grubb [28] described allotypy in human immunoglobulins. Allotypes are antigenic determinants on protein molecules (not necessarily immunoglobulins) which are inherited in a simple Mendelian manner. They

31

differ in individuals of the same species and in some instances have been shown to correlate with differences in amino acid sequence of the protein. Allotypes are detected using antibodies produced by immunizing an animal with immune complexes or immunoglobulin which has been obtained from another animal of the same species having immunoglobulin allotypes differing from those of the immunized animal. Several groups of allotypes (groups a, d and e) detected by immunological methods have been described for rabbit immunoglobulins both in the constant and variable regions of the H chains (Fig. 3.13).

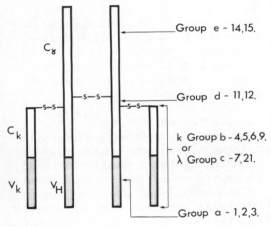

Fig. 3.13 Allotypes of rabbit IgG (after [29]).

Allotypes also occur on the light chains (groups b & c) but it is the presence of such markers in both C_H and V_H of the heavy chain which make them useful for studies into the genetic control of antibody synthesis. A rabbit H chain may carry an allotypic specificity from each of groups a, d, and e. It has been demonstrated that in a rabbit which is heterozygous at both the light chain groups (b group allotypes) and at the a group of the heavy chain, any one immunoglobulin molecule will carry only one of the two possible allelic markers of each group. Thus an animal which is genotypically a1, a3, b4, b6 will have immunoglobulin molecules which will have the specificities a1, b4; a1, b6; a3, b4 and a3, b6. Both H and L chains of each molecule have the same markers. This phenomenon is known as allotypic restriction. Of great interest was the surprising observation of Todd [30] that group a allotypes were present on both γ and μ chains and it has subsequently been shown that they are also present on α and ϵ chains. The significance of these observations (the 'Todd phenomenon') will be discussed later.

Table 3.3 The possible location of Gm and other markers in the homology regions of human IgG subclasses (after [30])

Subclass	Gm Type	Homology region Cγ1	Cγ2	Cγ3
IgG1	a^-f^+	f		non a
	$a^+x^+z^+$	z		a, x
IgG2	n^+		non g, n	non a
	n^-		non g	non a
IgG3	g^+		g	non a
	b^+		non g, b^1, s, t	non a, b^0, b^3, b^4, b^5, c^3, c^5
IgG4	—			$\gamma4$ non a

In human immunoglobulins, genetic markers (designated Gm) have been described on γ heavy chains. It has been shown that these markers are in the constant region of the heavy chain and are located in the Fc region of the molecule with the exception of Gm_f and Gm_z which are in the Fd region. It is thought that the subclass specific antigens are related to amino acid sequence differences. For example, it appears that there are two amino acid differences between residues 355 to 358 in the Fc fragments of IgG Gm(a) and IgG1 Gm(a⁻) proteins (see Table 3.4).

Table 3.4 Amino acid interchanges associated with allotype differences in subclasses of human IgG.

Subclass	Allotype	Residue Number	Amino Acid	
IgG1	Gm(a)	356,358	Asp	Leu
	Gm(a⁻)		Glu	Met
IgG1	Gm(f)	214	Arg	
	Gm(f⁻)		Lys	
IgG3	Gm(b)	436	Phe	
	Gm(g)		Tyr	
IgG3	Gm(b)	296	Phe	
	Gm(g)		Tyr	

A second system genetically closely linked to the Gm system has been described. This is the Am2 + marker on heavy chains of IgA2 proteins. An independently inherited marker in the constant region of human κ light chains — the Inv marker constitutes the third allotypic marker system of human immuno-globulins. A single amino acid substitution at residue 191 differentiates the Inv1 from the Inv3 determinant.

Human λ light chains exist in two forms which differ by one amino acid substitution at residue 190. In the Oz(+) subtype, lysine is at residue 190 and in the second type, the Oz(−) chains, the amino acid is arginine. These two types are present in all normal humans making it unlikely that they are allelic forms of a single gene locus. The subject of human immunoglobulin genetics has been recently reviewed [32].

Idiotypes It has been known for some time that immunization of a heterologous species with a myeloma protein produces an anti-antibody which, when absorbed with pooled human immunoglobulin still reacts specifically with the immunizing myeloma protein. Antibodies are directed towards individual anti-genic determinants present in the Fab part of the myeloma protein. 'Anti-antibodies' raised in homologous species of the *same* allotype as the immunizing immunoglobulin have been described as anti-idiotypic antibodies. These are directed towards determinants (idiotypes) located on the variable regions of the immunizing antibody molecules which are not present on the immunoglobulins of the immunized animal (i.e. are therefore recognized as 'foreign').

3.4 The biosynthesis of immunoglobulins

3.4.1 Cellular basis
Cellular immunologists have convincingly demonstrated that cells of the lymphoid system are responsible for immune reactions such as delayed hypersensitivity, graft rejection and antibody formation. The principal cells involved are the lymphocytes. These cells, although morphologically indistinguishable, can be classified by functional differences into two categories, one category which requires the thymus gland for development — the so-called thymus-dependent lymphocytes or T lymphocytes — and a second which develops independently of the thymus — the B-lymphocytes. (It should be noted that all lymphoid stem cells originate from the bone marrow.) The T-lymphocytes are responsible for the reactions of cell mediated immunity and the B-lymphocytes are precursors of cells which synthesise and secrete antibody — the plasma cells. While T-lymphocytes do not themselves produce antibody, they do co-operate with B-lymphocytes in antibody production, which has led to their description as 'helper' cells in this context. A third cell type — the macrophage — has also been impli-cated in the immune response. The major role of macrophages appears to be that of antigen handling, but there have also been reports that macrophages are able to transfer specific infor-mation to lymphocytes.

The classification of lymphocytes into two distinct immunologically competent types is based on experimental evidence in birds and rodents and on clinical observations in man. Removal of the thymus in birds or rodents markedly depresses the cell-mediated responses but has significantly less effect on humoral antibody responses. In birds, the removal of the bursa of Fabricius (a structure which is unique to birds) results in impaired humoral antibody responses but cell-mediated immune reactions are relatively unaffected. The nature of the equivalent to the avian bursa in other animals including man is unknown. The gut-associated lymphoid tissues such as appendix and tonsils have been suggested as bursa-equivalents, and circumstantial evidence in support of this suggestion is reviewed in [33].

T and B-lymphocytes can be distinguished on the basis of differences in surface antigens. In the mouse for example, T-lymphocytes have the characteristic θ antigen which is never present on antibody forming cells and B-lymphocytes have the mouse specific B-lymphocyte antigen (MBLA).

The clonal selection theory of Burnet [34] is widely accepted as a working hypothesis for antibody synthesis. This theory suggests that individual lymphocytes have the genetic capacity to make one, or possibly a small number of particular antibody specificities. The lymphocytes have, on their surface, immunoglobulin or immunoglobulin-like receptors. These receptors have the same specificity for antigen as the antibody which the cell can make when differentiated. Thus, when an antigen is presented to the lymphoid cells of an animal, cells with receptors which can react with the antigen will be stimulated to differentiate and will ultimately produce a clone of cells producing antibody with specificity towards the inducing antigen. Not all the cells differentiate into antibody forming

B cells (plasma cells) some become long-lived, antigen-reactive 'memory cells'. It is now clear that both B and T-lymphocytes can bind antigen via surface receptors and that cell selection as postulated by Burnet, does occur with both types. What is not clear, however, is the detailed immunochemical nature of those receptors, particularly T-lymphocyte receptors. The receptors of B-lymphocytes are immunoglobulin, as shown by techniques using specific antisera to various immunoglobulin determinants. Each cell has approximately $10^4 - 10^5$ immunoglobulin molecules on its surface. IgG, IgM, IgA and IgD receptors have been demonstrated and in the human, subclasses of IgG have been shown on B-lymphocyte cell surfaces. It is thought that the immunoglobulin receptors are oriented with the Fc regions towards the B-lymphocyte surface leaving the antibody binding sites free to react with the antigen. The nature of receptors on T-lymphocytes is a controversial issue and convincing information as to their immunoglobulin nature has yet to be provided. Indeed, it has been suggested that non-immuno-globulin receptors such as the products of immune response (I_r) genes, are involved in T-lymphocyte recognition of antigen. This discussion of such a wide field is of necessity very brief. However, the role of T and B-lymphocytes in immune reactions has been reviewed recently [35] from which several relevant references can be obtained.

3.4.2 Synthesis, assembly and secretion
Once antigen-induced selection, differentiation and proliferation of antibody-forming B-lymphocytes has occurred, antibody is produced and appears in the circulation. The genetic control of this process is not completely understood (see section 3.4.3). The biochemistry has been elegantly unravelled by Askonas and Williamson and others (see [36] for review and references) who have exploited the use of experimentally induced mouse myeloma tumors each making a unique myeloma protein.

It appears that immunoglobulin synthesis is achieved by plasma cells by the normal processes of protein synthesis. Heavy and light immunoglobulin polypeptide chains are synthesised on separate ribosomes, heavy chains are synthesised on polyribosomes consisting of 11−18 ribosomes with an ultracentrifuge sedimentation rate of 300S and light chains on polyribosomes of 200S consisting of 4−5 ribosomes. Light chains are rapidly released from the polyribosomes and enter an intracellular pool which is maintained at a constant size. Free H chains are not normally present in the cell. Heavy and light chain synthesis is normally balanced to result in the formation and secretion of completed molecules. The result of pulse labelling experiments with radioactive amino acids have shown that there is a gradient of radioactivity from the C-terminal to the N-terminal amino acids of both heavy [37] and light chains [38] which is consistent with the synthesis of the chains as a single unit from the N-terminal end.

Completed immunoglobulin molecules are held in their stable configuration by covalent and non-covalent bonds. Inter- and intra-chain disulphide bonds play an important part in this stabilization. It is suggested [36] that covalent interchain disulphide bond formation follows the non-covalent assembly of the chains into a stable quarternary structure. H−H and H−L disulphide bonds are normally produced and the order in which these are formed has been studied by pulse labelling of immunoglobulin secreting cells and subsequent analysis of the products by electrophoresis under dissociating conditions. Two groups of intermediates have been identified as shown in Fig. 3.14. The intermediates formed vary from species to species and within immunoglobulin classes as shown in Table 3.15.

The situation with the polymeric immunoglobulins IgM and IgA is particularly interesting.

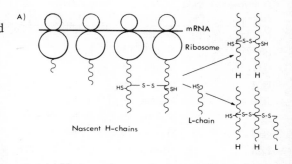

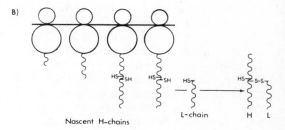

Fig. 3.14 Order of disulphide bond formation (a) H−H before H−L; (b) H−L before H−H.

It appears that the precursor of IgM in a mouse myeloma is the monomeric $H_2 L_2$ form (IgMs) and that no pentameric IgM is detectable inside the cell. Polymerization to give the pentameric IgM molecule probably occurs just before or at the time of secretion [39]. A similar situation exists with polymeric IgA.

Although immunoglobulins are glycoproteins containing relatively high levels of carbohydrate (particularly IgM and IgA) no function for these prosthetic groups has yet been established. The early suggestion that the addition of carbohydrate is a prequisite for secretion [39, 40] is still being debated.

An attractive model for the secretion of immunoglobulin has been suggested [41] and is

Table 3.5 Immunoglobulin disulphide bond formation (after [35]).

Immunoglobulin class	Species	Intermediate H.H−L	H−H	HL
IgG2a	Mouse	+	+	−
IgG2b	Mouse	+	+	+
IgG1	Mouse	+	+	−
IgM	Mouse	−	−	+
IgA	Mouse	−	+	−
IgG	Rabbit	−	−	+
IgG	Human	+	+	−
IgM	Human	−	−	+

essentially as follows: Immunoglobulin chains are synthesised and partially assembled on polyribosomes. Carbohydrate is added to the molecule in the rough endoplasmic reticulum. The chains enter the cisternae of the endoplasmic reticulum and the four-chain molecule is formed in the cisternal space. The completed molecule is transported to the Golgi complex where further carbohydrate is added. After this it is presumed that the molecule is contained in secretory vesicles prior to secretion.

3.4.3 The genetic control of immunoglobulin biosynthesis

The results of amino acid sequence analysis of many human light chains has revealed the existence of two distinct regions of the chain, the variable region V_L and the constant region C_L (see above). The existence of the V_L and C_L regions in light chains has led to the unique suggestion that the well-established 'one-gene-one polypeptide chain' concept does not hold, and that for these polypeptides two genes code for one polypeptide chain [43]. Analysis of H chain amino acid sequence data revealing similar constant and variable regions has resulted in the two gene-one polypeptide chain concept also being applied to these chains. More recently, the demonstration of three homology regions in

the constant part of human H chains together with the variable region [19] has led to the suggestion that perhaps four genes are involved in H chain synthesis.

Several observations lend support to the two gene-one polypeptide chain hypothesis; (a), The observation [30] that V_H region rabbit allotypes are shared by IgG, IgM, IgA and IgE (Todd phenomenon); (b), Examples of shared idiotypy — i.e. the presence of the same variable region marker on antibodies of different H chain classes — have been described including shared idiotypic determinants on both rabbit IgG and IgM anti-*Salmonella typhi* antibodies [44]; (c), Two myelomas IgG2κ and IgMκ in the same patient but made in different plasma cells have been shown to have identical amino acid sequences up to 34 residues from the N-terminus including the hypervariable region around residue 30 (See Fig. 3.11), and also shared idiotypic determinants whilst possessing different constant regions [45]. (d) in the human, a study of amino acid sequence data for both heavy and light chains suggests that separate genetic systems are involved for C and V region synthesis [46]. In light chains for example, it seems that C_λ and C_κ genes have exclusive V_λ and V_κ gene pools. Thus the single C_κ gene can be associated with any one of these V_κ subgroup genes and the two C_λ genes can be associated with any one of five V_λ subgroup genes. With heavy chains it seems that all V_H region genes belong to a single heavy chain group — consisting of four subgroups — which can be associated with any C_H region gene — See Table 3.6. If separate V and C region genes exist at different loci in the genome, the question is raised as to how they are combined to form a VC structural gene in the immunocompetent cells, such that a single mRNA specifying amino acid sequences for the complete chain is produced. Several theories have been proposed to explain how this could be achieved. One such theory [47] involves a somatic translocation mechanism. A circular

36

Table 3.6 Minimum genetic system for human immunoglobulin polypeptide chain genes (after [45]).

Chain	V-region subgroup genes	C region genes
κ	V_κ	κ
λ	$V_{\lambda\ I-V}$	λoz^+
		λoz^-
Heavy	$V_{H\ I-IV}$	$C\gamma 1, 2, 3, 4$
		$C\alpha 1, 2$
		$C\mu 1, 2$
		$C\delta 1, 2$
		$C\epsilon 1, 2$

episome-like DNA particle (coding for a single V sequence) is produced by intra-chromosomal translocation and is integrated into the DNA adjacent to the necessary C region gene. The resulting VC structural gene is then transcribed to form the necessary mRNA for polypeptide chain synthesis. This type of integration has a precedent in nature in that λ phage genome integrates into part of the host bacterial genome.

More recently, a copy-choice VC integration mechanism has been suggested in which a V_H gene is selected and repeatedly copied and integrated into the DNA adjacent to C_H genes (C_γ, C_μ etc.) on the same chromosome [48]. This takes into account both (i), several biological observations that individual cells can 'switch' from IgM to IgG antibody synthesis while retaining the same antibody specificity, and (ii), the occurrence of double myelomas in a single patient (described above) with identical V region sequences but different C regions.

One question which is still unresolved is what is the origin of antibody diversity? Since a mature animal can produce a large number of possible antibodies and such antibody specificity resides in the variable regions of the immunoglobulin chains, there are obviously very many V genes in the genome.

It is generally accepted that each antibody specificity reflects the number of variable regions which can be synthesised and that each V_H-V_L binding site is specific for one antigen. However, it has been recently pointed out [49] that the possibility of polyfunctional binding sites may have far reaching implications with respect to our theories of the genetic control of antibody production, particularly since such polyfunctional sites would represent a significant gene-saving mechanism. There are two theories which attempt to explain the origin of antibody diversity. The first — the so-called germ-line theory — suggests that a sufficient number of V genes is transmitted via the germ line such that combination of V_L and V_H gene products provides all the necessary binding sites for combination with a large number of antigens. The second, — the somatic mutation theory — suggests that a small number of V genes are transmitted via the germ-line and that, during the development of the individual, V gene diversity is achieved by random somatic mutation such that immunocompetent cells each express different specificities. These two theories have no shortage of supporters and supporting data and it is likely that the debate will continue for some time.

For detailed consideration of the problems of the genetic control of antibody production, the interested reader should consult references [45, 46 and 50].

References
[1] Tiselius, A. & Kabat, E.A. (1938), *Science* **87**, 416.
[2] *Methods in Immunology and Immunochemistry Volume I* (1967) *and Volume II* (1968), Edited by C.A. Williams & M.A. Chase, Academic Press, London and New York.
[3] Schultze, H.E. & Heremans, J.F. (1960), *Molecular Biology of Human Proteins*, Volume I, Elsevier, Amsterdam.
[4] Gill, T.J. III (1970), *Immunochemistry* **7**, 99.

[5] Farr, R.S. & Minden, P. (1968), *Ann. N.Y. Acad. Sci*, **154**, 107.

[6] Minden, P., Anthony, B.F. & Farr, R.S. (1969), *J. Immunol.* **102**, 832.

[7] Porter, R.R. (1959), *Biochem. J.* **73**, 119.

[8] Nisonoff, A., Wissler, F.C. & Lipman, L.N. (1960), *Science* **132**, 1770.

[9] Porter R.R. (1962), in *Basic Problems of Neoplastic Disease*, Ed. by Abellhorn & E. Hirschberg, Columbia Univ. Press, New York.

[10] Porter R.R. (October 1967), *Scientific American – The Structure of Antibodies*, p. 81.

[11] Valentine R.C. & Green N.M. (1967), *J. Mol. Biol.* **27**, 615.

[12] Stanworth, D.R. & Turner M.W. (1973). in *Handbook of Experimental Immunology*, 2nd Edition, D.M. Weir, Ed. Blackwell Scientific Publications, Oxford.

[13] Frangione, B., Milstein, C. & Pink, J.R.L. (1969), *Nature* **221**, 145.

[14] Grey H.M., Abel, C.A., Yount, W.J. & Kunkel, H.G. (1968), *J. Exp. Med.* **128**, 1223.

[15] Steward M.W. (1971), *Biochem. Biophys. Acta* **236**, 440.

[16] Small, P.A., Curry, J. & Waldman, R.H. (1971), *The Secretory Immunologic System*, 1969, U.S. Dept. Health, Education & Welfare, p. 13.

[17] Halpern, H.S. & Koshland, M.E. (1970), *Nature*, **228**, 1276.

[18] Putnam, F.W., Titani, K., Wikler, M. & Shinoda, T. (1967), *Cold Spring Harbor Symposium on Quantitative Biology*, Vol. 32, p. 9.

[19] Edelman, G.M., Cunningham, B.A., Gall, W.G., Gottlieb, P.D., Rutishauser, U. & Waxdall, M.J. (1969), *Proc. Nat. Acad. Sci. U.S.A.* **63**, 78.

[20] Edelman, G.M. & Gall, W.E. (1969), *Ann. Rev. Biochem.* **38**, 415.

[21] Edelman, G.M. (1971), *Proc. N.Y. Acad. Sci.* **190**, p. 5.

[22] Yoo, T.J., Roholt, O.A. & Pressman, D. (1967), *Cold Spring Harbor Symposium on Quantitative Biology*, Vol. 32, p. 117.

[23] Haber, E. & Richards, F. (1967), *Proc. Roy. Soc.* **166B**, 176.

[24] Cohn, M. (1971), *Proc. N.Y. Acad. Sci.* **190**, p. 529.

[25] Singer, S.J. & Doolittle, R.F. (1966), *Science*, **153**, 13.

[26] Krause, R.M. (1970), *Advanc. Immunol.* **16**, 1

[27] Oudin, J. (1956), *Compt. Rend.* **242**, 2606.

[28] Grubb, R. (1956), *Acta Path. Microbiol. Scand.* **39**, 195.

[29] Todd, C.W. (1972), *Fed. Proc.* **31**, 188.

[30] Todd. C.W. (1963), *Biochem. Biophys. Res. Commun.* **11**, 170.

[31] Natvig. J.B. & Turner, M.W. (1971), *Clin. Exp. Immunol.* **8**, 685.

[32] Natvig, J.B. & Kunkel, H.G. (1973), *Advanc. Immunol.* **16**, 1.

[33] Cooper, M.D. & Lawton, A.R. (1972), in *Contemporary Topics in Immunobiology*, Volume 1 (Hanna, M.G. ed.) Plenum Press, New York, p. 49.

[34] Burnet, F.M. (1957), *Austr. J. Sci.* **20**, 67; (1959) *The clonal selection theory of acquired immunity*. Cambridge Univ. Press.

[35] Raff, M.C. (1973), *Nature* **242**, 19.

[36] Bevan, M.J., Parkhouse, R.M.E., Williamson, A.R. & Askonas, B.A. (1972), in *Progress in Biophysics and Molecular Biology*, (Butler, J.A.V. and Noble, D. Eds.) Vol. **25**, p. 133.

[37] Fleischman, J. (1967), *Biochemistry* **6**, 1311.

[38] Lennox, E.S., Knopf, P.M., Munro, A.J. & Parkhouse, R.M.E. (1963), *Cold Spring Harbor Symposium on Quantitative Biology*. **32**, p. 249.

[39] Parkhouse, R.M.E. & Askonas, B.A. (1969), *Biochem. J.* **115**, 163.

[40] Eylar, E.M. (1966), *J. Theoret. Biol.* **10**, 89.

[41] Swenson, R.M. and Kern, M. (1967), *J. Biol. Chem.* **242**, 3242.

[42] Sherr, C.J., Schenkein, I. & Uhr, J.W. (1971), *Proc. N.Y. Acad. Sci.* **190**, p. 250.

[43] Dreyer, W.J. & Bennett, J.C. (1965), *Proc. Nat. Acad. Sci. U.S.* **54**, 864.

[44] Oudin, J. and Michel M. (1969), *J. Exp. Med.*, **130**, 619.

[45] Fudenberg, H.H., Pink, J.R.L., Stites, D.C. & Waney, A.C. (1972), *Basic Immunogenetics*, Oxford University Press.

[46] Pink, J.R.L., Wang, A.C. & Fudenberg, H.H. (1971), *Ann. Rev. Med.* **22**, 145.

[47] Gally, J.A. & Edelman, G.M. (1970), *Nature*, **227**, 341.

[48] Williamson, A.R. (1971), *Nature*, **231**, 359.

[49] Richards, F.F. & Konigsberg, W.H. (1973), *Immunochemistry*, **10**, 545.

[50] McDevitt, H.O. & Benacerraf, B. (1969), *Advanc. Immunol.* **11**, 31.

4 Antibody-antigen interaction

In order to study the antibody-antigen interaction it is generally necessary to determine in some way the free and bound forms of either antigen or antibody after they have interacted.

The simplest method for partitioning insoluble antibody-antigen complexes from soluble reactants is the precipitation reaction (a secondary test). For many years this was the only test available to immunochemists and detailed studies of this process have provided much information of the nature of antibody-antigen interactions. Arrhenius (1907) was the first to apply the Law of Mass Action to immunochemical reactions in his attempts to describe mathematically the immune precipitation reaction. We now know that this law does not apply to the complex secondary reactions involved in precipitate formation but this work is nevertheless, a landmark in the history of immunochemistry.

4.1 Precipitation reactions

The work of Arrhenius and those who followed him was seriously hampered by the fact that although immune precipitates could be measured, their actual composition could not be chemically quantitated since both antibody and antigen were proteins. For similar reasons the determination of antibody and antigens in the supernatant was not possible. This problem was overcome by Heidelberger and Kendall [1] by using pneumococcal polysaccharides as antigens which do not interfere with antibody nitrogen determinations. More recently, of course, the application of radioisotope techniques has eliminated these difficulties. However, using polysaccharide antigens, Heidelberger and his colleagues (reviewed in [2]) have described the generalized form of the immunological precipitation reaction which is shown in Fig. 4.1.

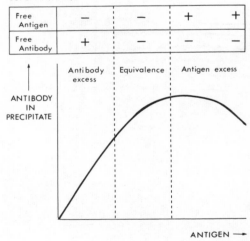

Fig. 4.1 The quantitative precipitation reaction.

As increasing amounts of antigen are added to a fixed amount of antibody, the quantity of antibody precipitated increases. After the addition of small amounts of antigen, some precipitate is formed and free antibody is detectable in the supernatant — this is the *antibody excess zone*. Here the ratio of antibody to antigen in the immune complex depends on the valency of the antigen. The addition of larger amounts of antigen results in increased precipitation until a point is reached where no free antibody or antigen is detectable in the supernatant. This is the *equivalence zone*. Marrack [3] hypothesised that at this point, optimal proportions of antibody and antigen form a continuous, stable antibody-antigen 'lattice' which precipitates. At high levels of antigen, free antigen appears in the supernatant and at the same time, precipitate formation is still maximal. This is the first stage of the *antigen excess zone*. At conditions of extreme antigen excess, the amount of precipitate is markedly reduced, due to the formation of soluble complexes. Solubilization results from the excess free antigen competing for the antibody sites in the precipitate with subsequent formation of soluble complexes with the molar composition $Ab_1 Ag_2$.

Both the quantity and quality (See 4.3) of antibody is important in determining whether a precipitate will be formed. Antigenic valency is also a critical factor since the formation of a lattice is impossible if the antigen is monovalent.

4.2 Agglutination reactions
The formation of a lattice with antibody and a multivalent antigen results in precipitation as discussed above. However, when antibody reacts with antigenic sites on the surface of particles such as those on red blood cells or bacteria, agglutination occurs. Inert particles such at latex, coated with antigen are also agglutinated by antibody (passive agglutination).

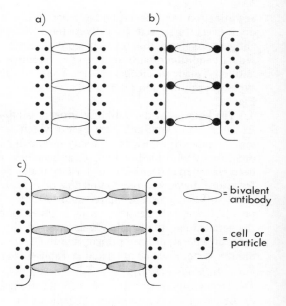

Fig. 4.2 Agglutination reactions. (a), active agglutination; (b) passive agglutination with antigen, (●) coated onto cell or particle; (c), Coombs test: agglutination by incomplete antibodies (shaded) only on addition of anti-γ-globulin (open).

Essentially what occurs is that sufficient antibody-antigen bonds are formed to overcome the natural repulsive charge effects of cells, which results in their aggregation or agglutination. As with precipitation reactions, the valency of the antigen and the nature of the antibody are important in agglutination reactions. Cells with few antigenic determinants will be less readily agglutinated than those with many determinants. The multivalent IgM antibody is, on a molecule to molecule basis, a more efficient agglutinating antibody than the divalent IgG. Univalent antibodies or incomplete antibodies (antibodies which do not agglutinate or precipitate antigen for physicochemical or structural reasons) can be demonstrated by the Coombs test. In this agglutination test, the antibodies react with, but do not agglutinate cells (or cells coated with antigen). Agglutination is produced by the subsequent addition of antibodies to the incomplete antibody, made in another species. These three types of agglutination reactions are shown in Fig. 4.2.

4.3 The kinetics of the antibody-antigen reaction

As described in section 3.2 the events which may or may not follow the primary interaction of antibody with the homologous antigen have been classified as secondary or tertiary manifestations. In view of the complexity of variables which influence these secondary and tertiary manifestations, studies attempting to investigate the detailed nature of antibody-antigen reactions have, in general, utilized primary binding techniques, some of which are listed in Table 4.1.

4.3.1 Antibody affinity

The term antibody affinity refers to the strength of the interaction between an antigenic determinant and the homologous antibody. In effect it is the summation of the attractive and repulsive forces described in section 4.4. Thus a high affinity antibody is one which forms a strong bond with the antigenic determinant to give an antibody antigen complex with a low tendency to dissociate. On the other hand, a low

Table 4.1 Quantitative primary binding tests

1. Equilibrium dialysis
2. Fluorescence quenching
3. Fluorescence enhancement
4. Fluorescence polarization
5. Separation of complexes from free antigen by
    (i) ammonium sulphate precipitation
    (ii) antiglobulin precipitation
    (iii) ultracentrifugation
    (iv) gel filtration
    (v) polyacrylamide disc electrophoresis
    (iv) adsorption of antigen onto charcoal, silica
6. Temperature jump method
7. Water extrusion methods.

affinity antibody forms a complex with antigen which requires less energy for dissociation. Thus the higher the affinity of the antibody, the greater will be the amount of antigen bound to antibody at equilibrium. Affinity is a thermodynamic measurement of the strength of the antibody-antigen interaction and is expressed either as the equilibrium constant K (with units of litres/mole) or as the standard free energy change $\Delta G°$(with units of k calories/mole). The quantitative relationship of the interaction between antibody and antigen at equilibrium is represented by the equation:

$$Ab + Ag \underset{k_d}{\overset{k_a}{\rightleftharpoons}} AbAg$$

where Ab represents free antibody, Ag free antigen, $AbAg$, the antibody-antigen complex, k_a and k_d the association and dissociation constant respectively.

The Law of Mass Action states that the rate of formation of complex is proportional to the concentration of the reactants. Thus the rate of association is equal to $k_a (Ab)(Ag)$, and the rate of dissociation is equal to $k_d (Ab\ Ag)$. At equilibrium the rates of association and dissociation are equal, thus:

$$k_a(Ab)(Ag) = k_d (AbAg)$$

$$\therefore \frac{k_a}{k_d} = K = \frac{(AbAg)}{(Ab)(Ag)} \qquad (4a)$$

where K is the equilibrium constant, also $\Delta G° = -RT \ln K$ where R is the gas constant and T the absolute temperature. Thus a high affinity antibody will have a more negative $\Delta G°$ value compared to that of a low affinity antibody.

At this point, a note of clarification is necessary. In the literature, the terms 'affinity' and 'avidity' are often used synonymously. Affinity is a thermodynamic expression of the primary binding energy of antibody for an antigenic determinant. Experimentally this term has its most precise application in monovalent hapten-anti hapten systems. Avidity on the other hand, although it depends in part on affinity, also involves factors such as antibody valency, antigen valency and other nonspecific factors associated with binding. For example, a multivalent IgM antibody whose binding sites have the same affinity for antigen as a bivalent IgG antibody, will have a greater avidity for a multivalent antigen than the IgG antibody. The IgM is a more avid antibody because its multiple binding sites give it a greater ability to bind the antigen. The avidity of an antibody is often expressed in terms of its ability to effect a biological antigen binding function, such as virus neutralisation. This clearly involves factors other than primary antibody-antigen binding. Thus affinity and avidity are not synonymous.

4.3.2 Derivation of equations for affinity calculation

Thermodynamic measurement of antibody affinity requires that the reactants — antigen and antibody — are pure and in solution. Ideally the reactants should be homogeneous with regard to antigenic determinants and binding sites. Such measurements with antibodies are complicated because of their heterogeneity and multivalency for antigen. However, in spite of these limitations, reasonably precise affinity measurements can be made with antibodies to a monovalent hapten. Affinity measurements with antibody-antigen systems which are less thermodynamically precise can be made but such determinations only provide relative affinity values, e.g. with antiprotein antibodies.

The equilibrium constant K, or affinity, of isolated specific anti-hapten antibody (see section 3.1) can be determined experimentally by measurement of free hapten and antibody bound hapten at equilibrium over a range of hapten concentrations (See Table 4.1 and Section 4.3.3 below). The following is a brief outline of the derivation of equations frequently used for affinity calculations using the data from such experiments. Detailed derivations can be obtained from references [5] and [6].

From the Law of Mass Action the following form of the Langmuir adsorption isotherm may be derived:

$$\frac{(AbAg)}{(Ab)} = r = \frac{nK(Ag)}{1 + K(Ag)} \qquad (4b)$$

Where r = moles hapten bound per mole of antibody present, $(AbAg)$ = bound antibody concentration, (Ab) free antibody concentration, (Ag) free hapten concentration, n = antibody valence, K = equilibrium constant. From which:

$$\frac{r}{(Ag)} = nK - rK \qquad (4c)$$

Thus a plot of $r/(Ag)$ versus r (Scatchard Plot) for a range of antigen concentrations allows n, the antibody valence and K to be obtained (Figure 4.3).

This equation is frequently used to obtain values for the intrinsic association constant K_0 in systems involving a divalent antibody ($n = 2$) and a monovalent hapten. When half the antibody sites are bound (i.e. $r = 1$) then

$$\frac{r}{(Ag)} = nK - rK$$

becomes

$$\frac{1}{(Ag)} = 2K - K = K_0$$

Thus K_0 is equal to the reciprocal of the free hapten concentration at equilibrium when half the antibody sites are bound to hapten.

An alternative affinity equation can be obtained from either equation 4b or 4c:-

$$\frac{1}{r} = \frac{1}{n} \cdot \frac{1}{Ag} \cdot \frac{1}{K} + \frac{1}{n} \qquad (4d)$$

43

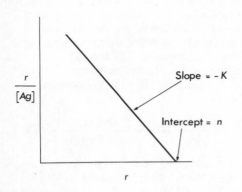

Fig. 4.3 Scatchard plot of ideal antibody-antigen binding.

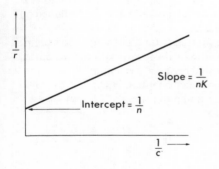

Fig. 4.4 Langmuir plot of ideal antibody-antigen binding.

A plot of $1/r$ versus $1/Ag$ (Langmuir plot) allows both antibody valence (n) and affinity K to be derived (Fig. 4.4). Both the Scatchard and Langmuir equations should give rise to straight line plots. However, with most antibodies-even when isolated and purified, there

is deviation from linearity. The reasons for this deviation are complex but it is basically due to the heterogeneity of antibody. Not all antibody molecules in an antibody population have the same affinity for the hapten. This deviation makes affinity determination using these equations difficult. Various mathematical techniques have been used to overcome this problem. The distribution of antibodies of various affinities within an antibody population is assumed to be describable in terms of a Gaussian or Sipsian function. By using the logarithmic transformation of the Sips equation [4,7]

$$\frac{r}{n} = \frac{(K_0 Ag)^a}{1 + (K_0 Ag)^a} \qquad (4e)$$

The following equation is obtained:-

$$\log \frac{r}{n-r} = a \log K_0 + a \log (Ag) \qquad (4f)$$

where a = heterogeneity index. Therefore, in a plot of $\log r/n - r$ versus $\log (Ag)$ where

$$\log \frac{r}{n-r} = 0, \text{ then } K_0 = \frac{1}{(Ag)}.$$

K_0 determined in this way is thus the peak of a presumed normal distribution curve. The heterogeneity index, a, is given by the slope of the line. (Fig. 4.5).

Thus in this way, the average intrinsic association constant K_0 and the heterogeniety index can be calculated. As the heterogeneity index approaches 1 the antibody population approaches homogeneity with regard to association constants.

In all that has been described so far, it is assumed that the antibody is pure and the amount present is known accurately. These calculations also require a knowledge of the valence of the antibody. In situations where isolation and purification of antibody is not possible or not desirable, calculation of K can be made with respect to total antibody binding

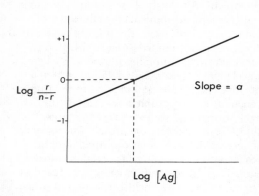

Fig. 4.5 Sips plot of antibody-antigen binding.

sites (Ab_t) rather than to antibody concentration and valence [8]. Thus equation (4b) becomes:-

$$\frac{b}{(Ab_t)} = \frac{K(Ag)}{1 + K(Ag)}$$

from which

$$\frac{1}{b} = \frac{1}{Ab_t} \times \frac{1}{Ag} \times \frac{1}{K} + \frac{1}{Ab_t} \qquad (4g)$$

Where b = antibody bound antigen and (Ag) free antigen. Thus measurement of bound and free antigen over a range of antigen concentrations and plotting the data according to equation 4g makes the determination of Ab_t (total antibody binding sites) possible i.e. when $1/(Ag) = 0$, then $1/b = 1/Ab_t$.

Affinity and heterogeneity index can be determined by substituting b for r and Ab_t for n in Equation (4f) [9].

4.3.3 Methods of affinity measurement

Basically, the measurement of antibody affinity depends upon the determination of free and antibody-bound antigen at equilibrium. Because of antibody heterogeneity such

determinations are usually carried over a range of antigen concentrations. This requires the separation of bound and free antigen either by a dialysis membrane, selective precipitation, gel filtration or by techniques which do not dissociate the bound antigen. Other methods utilize the alteration of some property of the antibody or antigen such as changes in fluorescence properties. Recently, techniques which utilize other physical changes which occur when antibody and antigen form a complex such as the measurement of changes in temperature and of volume (due to water extrusion) have been applied to affinity measurement (See Table 4.1). The most commonly used techniques will be briefly described.

Equilibrium dialysis This technique is widely accepted as the standard method of affinity measurement [10]. A dialysis membrane is used to partition antibody-bound hapten and free hapten. Antibody solution (purified antibody or immunoglobulin fraction of serum) is placed on one side and radioactive hapten on the other side of a dialysis membrane which allows the hapten to diffuse through it, but not the antibody. With time, hapten diffuses into the antibody compartment and some binds to the antibody. Equilibrium is eventually achieved when the free hapten concentration is the same on both sides of the membrane (Fig. 4.6). The radioactivity inside the antibody compartment represents bound and free hapten and that outside represents free hapten. Thus by subtraction, the amount of bound hapten is obtained. This process is repeated for several hapten concentrations using the same antibody concentration. The affinity of the antibody may then be calculated from the data by the methods described above.

Ammonium sulphate precipitation In this technique, the insolubility of antibody and hence antibody-hapten complexes in 50 per cent

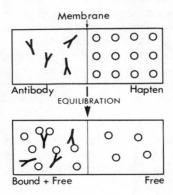

Membrane

Antibody | Hapten
EQUILIBRATION

Bound + Free | Free

Fig. 4.6 Diagram of equilibrium dialysis.

saturated ammonium sulphate is used [11].
Bound and free radioactive hapten concentrations can be readily determined by counting the precipitates and supernatants after precipitation with ammonium sulphate. This technique has been used for affinity measurement [9, 12] and the results obtained compare reasonably well with those determined by equilibrium dialysis [12]. It is ideal for rapid estimations of affinity and has the advantage of not requiring purified antibody. Whole serum can be used as a source of antibody. This method has also been applied to the measurement of the relative affinity of antibodies to protein antigens [9, 13]. However, in systems other than those involving hapten antigens, application is limited to those antigens which are soluble in 50% saturated ammonium sulphate.

Fluorescence quenching A molecule fluoresces when it absorbs light of one wavelength and then dissipates the absorbed energy by the emission of light at a longer wavelength.

Proteins fluoresce when irradiated with ultraviolet light. Although phenylalanine, tyrosine and tryptophan amino acid residues are all potentially fluorescent, the tryptophan residues make the major contribution to this fluorescence. Purified antibodies irradiated by light of wavelength between 280–295 nm emit light of wavelength 330–350 nm due to the fluorescence of their tryptophan residues. If this excitation energy is transferred to a nonfluorescent molecule the protein fluorescence is decreased. Thus when a purified antibody reacts with a hapten having certain fluorescence properties, the excitation energy produced on irradiation with u.v. light is transferred to the bound non-fluorescent hapten and is dissipated by non-fluorescent processes resulting in decreased or quenched antibody fluorescence. The method of fluorescence quenching was first described by Velick *et al* [14] using antibodies to the 2, 4 dinitrophenyl (DNP) group. The hapten DNP-lysine absorbs light maximally at 360 nm, and its absorption spectrum overlaps the antibody emission spectrum (Fig. 4.7) and is thus particularly suited to the study of antibody fluorescence quenching. The technique is quite straightforward. The maximum quenching (Q max) which can be obtained with all antibody sites occupied by hapten is first determined (up to 80% is possible). Then, assuming a linear relationship between quenching and number of antibody sites bound, the number of antibody sites bound at any given hapten concentration can be readily determined, and the antibody affinity calculated.

The method has the advantage of requiring small amounts of antibody but is limited to highly purified antibodies to haptens with the necessary spectral properties.

Fluorescence enhancement Changes in *hapten* fluorescence as a result of binding to antibody have been utilized for antibody affinity measurement. With certain fluorescent haptens,

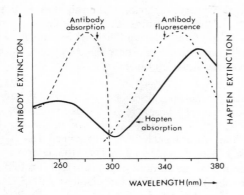

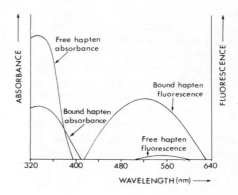

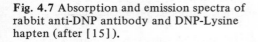

Fig. 4.7 Absorption and emission spectra of rabbit anti-DNP antibody and DNP-Lysine hapten (after [15]).

Fig. 4.8 Absorption and emission spectra of free and antibody-bound DANS-lysine (after [15]).

combination with antibody results in diminution of protein fluorescence but instead of the transferred excitation energy from the protein typtophan being dissipated, (as in the case with non-fluorescent haptens) the fluorescent hapten absorbs the energy and shows an increased fluorescence. This is known as fluorescence enhancement, and this property of certain haptens has been utilized for antibody affinity determinations. It has the distinct advantage of not requiring purified antibody since the fluorescence properties of the hapten and not those of the antibody are being measured.

An example of a molecule with such fluorescence properties is the dimethylamino-naphthalene-sulphonamido (DANS) group [14, 15]. This has an absorption maximum where tryptophan fluorescence is maximum and an absorption minimum where protein absorbs maximally. Maximum fluorescence is emitted at 520 nm where proteins do not fluoresce. Thus when rabbit antibodies react

with DANS-lysine, the fluorescence of the ligand is raised by 25–30 fold [15, 16] (See Fig. 4.8). This increase in fluorescence is related to the number of hapten molecules bound and can therefore be used to quantitate bound and free hapten at equilibrium for affinity determination. It is particularly useful for measuring antibodies of low affinity. For example, it has been used for demonstrating hapten binding by free light chains (See Fig. 3.10) which are of very low affinity.

Fluorescence polarization The fluorescent emission from a small molecule is not normally polarized because the molecules are randomly orientated during the short time interval between excitation and emission. The amount of rotation of a molecule as a result of rotatory Brownian motion decreases as molecular size increases. Thus, when a fluorescent molecule reacts with an antibody molecule, the size is obviously increased and the rotatory movement is restricted. The process of random orientation of the molecules in this situation is slower than for the free fluorescent molecule and this results

47

in the polarization of the fluorescent emission. The extent of flourescence polarization can be used to quantitate bound and free antigen and facilitate affinity determinations [17]. This method is applicable to the study of haptens and fluorescent labelled protein antigens and their interaction with the corresponding antibodies. The common labelling reagents for protein antigen studies are fluorescein isothiocyanate and dimethylaminonaphthalene sulphonyl chloride. The method is subject to certain problems particularly with larger antigens and is appraised by Parker in reference [15].

Other methods Several other methods for affinity determination are available including the use of the ultracentrifuge to quantitate the amount of bound and free antigen. The ultracentrifuge has been used to measure the affinity of rheumatoid factors for human IgG [18]. Rheumatoid factors are present in the serum of patients with rheumatoid arthritis, and are antibodies to immunoglobulins ('antiglobulins') which react with Fc antigenic determinants on the patients own IgG.

The use of gel filtration to provide antigen binding data for antibody affinity calculations has been described [19]. In this method, Sephadex beads (cross-linked dextran) of carefully chosen sizes are used to partition antibody bound antigen and free antigen on the basis of their size. Larger molecules (e.g. the antibody-antigen complex) are excluded from the beads whereas smaller molecules (i.e. free antigen) are able to enter the beads. This method has recently been applied to the measurement of the affinity of rheumatoid factors for isolated fragments of human IgG. These fragments (pF_c^-) bear the antigenic determinants to which the rheumatoid factor antibody activity is directed [20].

Measurement of the rate of dissociation of antibody-^{125}I-labelled antigen complexes in the presence of excess unlabelled antigen has been used to estimate the avidity of antibodies. In this case, high avidity antibodies have the faster association rates. The equilibrium constant K, can be calculated from these values, since $K = ka/kd$ (see equation (4a)).

All the methods discussed so far have applied to serum antibodies. A technique for measuring the avidity of antibodies at the level of the antibody forming cell has recently been described [22]. The method involves the determination of the amount of free antigen (protein or hapten) which will inhibit plaque-forming cells in the Jerne technique [23]. High affinity antibody producing cells require less free antigen to inhibit haemolytic plaque formation than do low affinity antibody producing cells.

4.4 The intermolecular forces involved in antibody-antigen interactions

The intermolecular forces which contribute to the stabilization of the antibody-antigen complex are the same as those involved in the stabilization of the configuration of proteins and other macromolecules. A brief account of these forces will be given here since they are fundamental to the specificity of the antibody-antigen interaction. Also qualitative measurements of the antibody-antigen interaction represent a summation of such intermolecular interactions. Detailed physico-chemical and mathematical consideration of these forces can be obtained from any physical chemistry text book.

4.4.1 Hydrogen bonding

Hydrogen bonding results from the interaction of an H atom covalently linked to an electronegative atom with the unshared electron pair of another electronegative atom. In antibody-antigen interactions, amino or hydroxyl groups are the major hydrogen donors. The following are examples of H bonds:-

the valence of IgM is very much influenced by the size of the antigen used [32]. The observed IgM anti-dextran valence varies from 10 for dextran of molecular weight 342, to 5 for dextrans of molecular weight 7 000–237 000. For dextrans of molecular weight 1.87×10^6 the observed valence is 2.3. These results clearly indicate that steric hindrance plays a vital role in determining the valence of IgM for an antigen.

The maturation phenomenon has been described for several antigens, usually after immunization in adjuvant. However, when human serum albumin is injected without adjuvants, maturation occurs but subsequently the affinity of serum antibody falls. This has been demonstrated in both rabbits [33] and mice [34]. These observations are difficult to reconcile with the selection theory but it is possible that in the absence of adjuvant (which in the case of Freund's complete adjuvant provides an antigen depot with continuous slow release of antigen over long periods), the decrease in affinity may be due to gradual death of short-lived high affinity antibody producing cells.

Since antibodies are multivalent, the question has been asked as to what is the functional significance of such multivalence. It has been known for some time that hapten-conjugated bacteriophage can be neutralized by anti-hapten antibody [35]. Work on the neutralization of DNP-conjugated bacteriophage $\phi \times 174$ by anti DNP antibodies [35] has provided convincing evidence that there is a greater energy of interaction between a multivalent antibody and a polyvalent antigen than between a monovalent antibody and polyvalent antigen. With the DNP-bacteriophage-anti DNP antibody system, the equilibrium constant of each antibody binding site for DNP-lysine (intrinsic affinity) can be determined by equilibrium dialysis. Also, kinetic studies of the neutralization of bacteriophage bearing multiple DNP groups by anti DNP allow calculation of equilibrium constants (functional affinity) in a polyvalent system. IgG anti DNP antibodies (divalent) have an intrinsic affinity for DNP-lysine of 10^7 litres/mole, and enhancement due to divalency of 10^3-fold. With IgM anti-DNP antibodies, intrinsic affinity was $10^4 - 10^5$ litres/mole whereas functional affinity was greater than 10^{11} litres/mole which represents an enhancement due to multivalency of 10^6-fold. These authors suggested that this represents multivalent IgM attachment to the conjugated phage via at least three of its binding sites. Similar work on DNP-T_4 bacteriophage [37] has provided confirmation of the concept that the neutralizing power of an antibody depends not only on concentration of antibody but also is a function of affinity, valence and molecular conformation. This enhancement of affinity due to multivalency represents a considerable advantage to the immune system in that considerably lower levels of multivalent antibody are required to provide an effective immune response than would be necessary with monovalent antibody. Multivalency may also be of significance in antigen stimulation of receptors on antigen sensitive cells particularly where IgM receptors are involved. Thus IgM receptors of low intrinsic affinity may bind antigen with high functional affinity and stimulate the cell to produce low affinity IgM. Cells with IgG receptors of high intrinsic affinity but similar functional affinity would also be stimulated which may explain the common observation that IgM antibodies seem to have lower affinity that IgG antibodies present in the serum at the same time.

Differences in antibody affinity produce marked differences in the biological activity of antibodies. For example, equal amounts of either high or low affinity antibody when passively transferred intravenously into recipient mice show marked differences in the immune elimination of ^{125}I-labelled antigen. High affinity

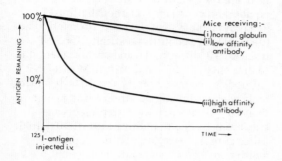

Fig. 4.9 Elimination of antigen by mice receiving passively transferred antibody of high or low affinity (after [38]).

antibody achieves greater elimination of antigen than does low affinity antibody, as shown in Fig. 4.9. The data shown in Table 4.1 show that complement fixation and passive cutaneous anaphyiaxis reactions are markedly affected by differences in antibody affinity.

Table 4.1 The effect of antibody affinity on the activity of antibodies (data from [39])

	Antibody preparation	
	A	B
Affinity, litres/mole	1×10^7	$1 \cdot 1 \times 10^6$
Antibody required for + ve PCA (μg/ml)	$31 \cdot 3 - 62 \cdot 5$	> 500
Conc.^{n} for complement fixation (2 units):		
Antibody (μg/ml)	$2 \cdot 10$	$8 \cdot 30$
Antigen (μg/ml)	$0 \cdot 03$	$0 \cdot 08$

Thus, high affinity antibody is far more efficient in complement fixation and passive cutaneous anaphylaxis reactions than is antibody with a 10-fold lower affinity.

It is hoped that the examples cited in this section have served to illustrate that antibody affinity is of critical importance in the immune response.

References
[1] Heidelberger, M. and Kendall, F.E. (1929), *J. Exp. Med.*, **50**, 809.
[2] Heidelberger, M. (1939), *Bacteriol, Rev.* **3**, 49.
[3] Marrack, J.R. (1938), *The Chemistry of Antigens and Antibodies*, H.M.S.O., London.
[4] Karush, F. (1962), *Advanc. Immunol.* **2**, 1.
[5] Day, E.D. (1972), *Advanced Immunochemistry*, Williams & Wilkins, Baltimore, p. 181
[6] Pinckard, R.N. & Weir, D.M. (1973), in *Handbook of Experimental Immunology*, Second Edition, (D.M. Weir, Ed), Blackwell Scientific Publications, Oxford, p. 16, Vol. **1**.
[7] Sips, R. (1948), *J. Chem. Phys.* **16**, 490.
[8] Nisonoff, A. & Pressman, D. (1958), *J. Immunol.* **80**, 417.
[9] Steward, M.W. & Petty, R.E. (1972), *Immunology*, **22**, 747.
[10] Eisen, H.N. (1964), *Methods in Medical Research*, **10**, 106.
[11] Farr, R.S. (1958), *J. Infect. Dis.* **103**, 239.
[12] Stupp, V., Yoshida, T. & Paul, W.E. (1969), *J. Immunol.*, **103**, 625.
[13] Steward, M.W. & Petty, R.E. (1972), *Immunology*, **23**, 881.
[14] Velick, S.F., Parker, C.W. & Eisen, H.N. (1960), *Proc. Nat. Acad. Sci.*, (Wash), **46**, 1470.
[15] Parker, C.W. (1973), in *Handbook of Experimental Immunology*, Second Edition, (D.M. Weir, Ed). Blackwell Scientific Publications, Oxford, p. 14, Vol. **1**.
[16] Parker, C.W., Yoo, T.J., Johnson, M.C. and Godt, S.M. (1967), *Biochemistry*, **6**, 3408.
[17] Dandliker, W.B., Schapiro, H.C., Meduski, J.W., Alonso, R., Feigen, G.A. & Hamrick, J.R. Jnr. (1964), *Immunochemistry*, **1**, 165.
[18] Normansell, D.E. (1970), *Immunochemistry*, **7**, 787.
[19] Stone, M.J. & Metzger, H. (1969), *J. Biol.*

Chem., **243**, 5049.

[20] Steward, M.W., Turner, M.W., Natvig, J.B. & Gaarder, P.I. (1973), *Clin. Exp. Immunol.*, **15**, 145.

[21] Talmage, D.W. (1960), *J. Infect. Dis.* **107**, 115.

[22] Andersson, B. (1970), *J. Exp. Med.* **132**, 77.

[23] Jerne, N.K. & Nordin, A.A. (1963), *Science*, **140**, 405.

[24] Karush, F. (1970), *Ann. N.Y. Acad. Sci.* **169**, 56.

[25] Eisen, H.N. & Siskind, G.W. (1964), *Biochemistry*, **3**, 996.

[26] Pressman, D., Roholt, D.A. & Grossberg, A.L. (1970), *Ann. N.Y. Acad. Sci.* **169**, 65.

[27] Werblin, T.P. & Siskind, G.W. (1972), *Immunochemistry*, **9**, 987.

[28] Siskind, G.W. & Benacerraf, B. (1969), *Advanc. Immunol.* **10**, 1.

[29] Werblin, T.P. & Siskind, G.W. (1972), *Transplant Reviews*, **8**, 104.

[30] Jerne, N.K. (1951), *Acta. Pathol. Microbiol. Scand.* Supp. **87**, 1.

[31] Steiner, L.A. & Eisen, H.N. (1967), *J. Exp. Med.* **126**, 1161.

[32] Edberg, S.C., Bronson, P.M. & Vanoss, C.J. (1972), *Immunochemistry*, **9**, 273.

[33] Urbain, J. Van Acker, A. Vos-Cloetens, C.H. & Urbain-Vansanten, G. (1972), *Immunochemistry*, **9**, 121.

[34] Petty, R.E., Steward, M.W. & Soothill, J.F. (1972), *Clin. Exp. Immunol.*, **12**, 231.

[35] Makela, O. (1966), *Immunology*, **10**, 81.

[36] Hornick, C.L. & Karush, F. (1972), *Immunochemistry*, **9**, 325.

[37] Blank, S.E., Leslie, G.A. & Clem, L.W. (1972), *J. Immunol.*, **108**, 665.

[38] Alpers, J.H., Steward, M.W. & Soothill, J.F. (1972), *Clin. Exp. Immunol.* **12**, 121.

[39] Fauci, A.S., Frank, M.M. & Johnson, J.J. (1970), *J. Immunol.* **105**, 215.

5 Biological activities of antibodies

In addition to the reaction with antigen which has been discussed earlier, immunoglobulins have many other biological activities. The antigen binding activity of antibodies is associated with the variable regions at the N-terminus of both heavy and light chains. The other biological activities of antibodies are associated with the Fc region of the heavy chains of certain immunoglobulin molecules. Some of these properties are only expressed when the antibody reacts with antigen. It has been suggested that this reaction results in an 'opening up' of the hinge region of the antibody molecule and initiates conformational changes in the Fc region which activate the biological properties characteristic for that particular immunoglobulin class or subclass. These properties differ within the various immunoglobulin classes and subclasses and are shown in Tables 5.1 and 5.2.

IgG is quantitatively the most important serum immunoglobulin in the human and is distributed almost equally between the intra- and extravascular fluids. Its major function is to neutralize viruses and bacterial toxins and bind to and opsonize bacteria (i.e. enhance their phagocytosis and elimination). IgG is the only immunoglobulin able to cross the placenta in the human and is thus a major defence mechanism against infection in the early part of a baby's life. The four subclasses of IgG differ in their biological properties (Table 5.2) particularly in complement fixing ability. IgG3 is the most efficient at complement fixation followed by IgG1 then IgG2 IgG4 does not fix complement. Although IgA is present in significant levels in the serum and has demonstrable antibody activity, it is in colostrum, saliva, tears, gastro-intestinal and respiratory tract secretions that this immunoglobulin is most important. In secretions, IgA is present as a dimer associated with the secretory component (see section 3.3.2) and is thought to provide an immunological barrier against micro-organisms by bathing the exposed mucosal surfaces [3].

IgM antibodies, as discussed in Chapter 4, are polyvalent which gives them a high functional affinity for multivalent antigens. This property, together with their effectiveness in agglutination, complement fixation, cytolysis, and predominant intravascular localization, indicates that IgM antibodies are particularly important in dealing with multivalent antigens such as bacteria and viruses infecting the blood stream.

Some antibody activity has been demonstrated in the IgD class of immunoglobulins such as anti-penicillin and antidiphtheria toxoid activity but the general biological function of these immunoglobulins is unknown.

IgE is present in the serum in extremely low concentrations and elevated levels are characteristically found in the serum of hay fever and asthma patients. Antibodies of this class can bind firmly to mast cells independent of any reaction with antigen. If an appropriate antigen (allergen) subsequently enters the host and reacts with the tissue fixed IgE antibody, a

Table 5.1 Biological properties of human immunoglobulins (after [1]).

Class	Serum conc. (mg/ml) mean & range	Intravascular distribution (%)	Half life (days)	Complement fixation	Placental transmission	Fixation to mast cells in human skin	Antibody activity
IgG	13·2 (7·5–22·1)	45	23·0	Yes	Yes	No	Major antiviral antibacterial and antitoxin activity in serum.
IgA (Serum)	1·6 (0·5–3·4)	42	5·8	No*	No	No	Antiviral and antibacterial activity.
IgA (Secretions)	—	—	—	No	No	No	Major antiviral and antibacterial activity in secretions.
IgM	0·9 (0·2–2·8)	76	5·1	Yes	No	No	Antipolysaccharide activity. Good agglutinator.
IgD	0·1 (<0·1–0·5)	75	2·8	No	No	No	Some antibody activities but major function unknown.
IgE	0·00033 (0·0001–0·0013)	51	2·3	No	No	Yes	Reaginic antibodies. Raised levels in parasitic infections.

* IgA can activate the alternate pathway of complement fixation.

Table 5.2 Biological activities of human IgG subclasses (after [1]).

IgG Subclass	Incidence (%)	Half life (days)	Complement (C1q) fixation	Placental transmission	Heterologous skin fixation	Opsonic activity	Specificity for mono-nuclear cells
1	70	15–19	++	+	+	+	+
2	18	24	+	+	0	0	0
3	8	?	+++	+	+	+	+
4	3	?	0	+	+	0	0

chain of events is triggered. The mast cells degranulate, vasoactive amines (e.g. histamine) are released and subsequent clinical symptoms of immediate hypersensitivity or 'allergy' such as sneezing and urticaria are produced. Current ideas on the mechanisms involved in immediate hypersensitivity can be obtained from reference [3].

The biological activities of immunoglobulins mentioned so far will be described briefly below.

5.1 Complement fixation

Complement is a complex biological system of nine protein components (C1–C9) the first of which, when activated by immune complexes, becomes able to activate the next component in the sequence which can itself activate the next component and so on, thus producing a 'cascade' effect. The activation of this system has profound effects on biological membranes and the terminal components have the capacity to cause cell death by punching holes through the membrane on which they are fixed. As well as potentiating cell lysis, activation of the complement system also promotes chemotaxis – the attraction of polymorphonuclear phagocytes to the site of the antibody: antigen reaction – and other aspects of inflammation such as increased vascular permeability. These properties of complement activation are posessed by breakdown or fusion products of the activated complement proteins.

The chemistry of this process has been studied in great detail during the last few years and methods are available for separation of the proteins involved (See [4, 5] for references).

The initial step in the activation of the complement sequence by antibody-antigen complexes is the binding of C1 to active sites on the Fc of the antibody which have been produced as a result of immune complex formation. As discussed above, immunoglobulin classes and subclasses differ in their ability to bind complement. It appears that for haemolytic activity a minimum of two adjacent IgG antibody molecules bound to the antigen is required to bind the C1 recognition unit whereas for IgM with multiple Fc regions, the requirement is for only one molecule. The C1 recognition unit consists of three subunit types:- C1q, C1r and C1s which are present in the ratio $1:2:4$ [4], and the reaction with the altered antibody occurs through the C1q component which is polyvalent, and can bind 5 IgG molecules. This binding appears to involve a site on the C_H2 homology region of the IgG. This binding results in C1r activating C1s. The active form of C1s is an enzyme the substrates of which are components C4 and C2. It first catalyses the binding of C4 to the cell and then the binding of C2 to the bound C4. This complex ($C\overline{42}$) is termed C3 convertase which has C3 as its substrate. At this stage two events occur as a result of C3 convertase activity on C3 [1]. Fragments of C3 called C3a are released. These have anaphylatoxin (histamine release) activity and are also chemotactic for polymorphonuclear phagocytes [11]. The major fragment of C3, – called C3b – is transferred to the target cell membrane, and is recognized by the C3 binding sites of macrophages leading to immune adherence and subsequent phagocytosis. C3b also modifies the $C\overline{42}$ enzyme to produce the $C\overline{423}$ enzyme. This acts on C5 which then interacts with C6 and C7 resulting in the binding of $C\overline{567}$ to the membrane. Also at this stage, further fragments with chemotactic and anaphylatoxin activity are produced. Finally C8 and C9 become attached to the membrane and a lesion (approx. 100 Å in diameter) is produced by an, at present, unknown mechanism. The C8 can bind up to six C9 molecules. This latter point is an example of how the effect of the complement is amplified. Since enzymes which react with several substrate molecules are produced at each stage in the complement sequence it can be seen that each activated complement component can activate several molecules of the next component and so on, resulting in a considerable amplification of the effect of the complement sequence. This pathway is known as the classical complement pathway and is represented schematically in Fig. 5.1. Another complement activating mechanism (the 'alternative' or 'by-pass' pathway) has been recently described in which the C1, C2, and C4 are by-passed and the C3 is activated directly by a C3 activator [6]. A component of serum, the C3 proactivator (C3PA) is activated by one of several substances such as inulin, endotoxins and certain aggregated immunoglobulins (including aggregated IgA1 and IgA2 myeloma proteins) to produce two substances. One of these substances can cleave C3 into C3a and C3b and so initiate the activation of components C3–C9 and is called the C3 activator. It is possible that IgA antibodies may utilize this alternate pathway. IgG1, 2 & 3 antibodies appear to utilize both pathways whilst IgM operates only via the classical pathway [4].

Obviously, such a potent biological system as complement fixation must be subject to strict control. Homeostatic control of the pathway is achieved at various stages. For example, C1 inhibitor limits the action of activated C1 on C4 and C2; $C\overline{42}$ is unstable and this limits the activity of C3 convertase; C3b inactivator (KAF) inhibits the haemolytic activity of bound C3. Other activators and inhibitors are currently being studied.

Detailed information on complement chemistry and activation can be obtained from references [4–8]. The subject has been reviewed recently [9].

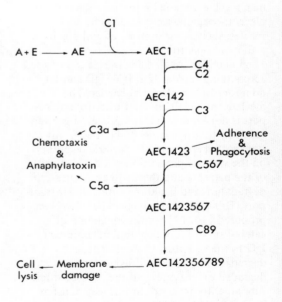

Fig. 5.1 Complement activation pathway.

5.2 Other biological properties of antibodies

In addition to participating in the activation of complement, antibodies also have several other biological properties associated with structures in the Fc region. These include regulation of the placental transfer and control of catabolism, binding to macrophages and mast cells and reactivity with rheumatoid factors (anti-immunoglobulin antibodies).

Although very young animals can make antibodies, they normally depend upon transferred immunoglobulins from their mother either at the foetal or neonatal stage. Animals differ in the way this is achieved. Some, such as the pig, horse, sheep, goat and cow receive maternal immunoglobulins entirely in the post-natal period via the colostrum. Others such as rabbit, guinea-pig, monkey and also man receive maternal immunoglobulins by placental or yolk-sac transmission. In some species, such as the mouse, rat and dog both routes are operating.

In man, IgG of all subclasses is transported across the placenta. IgA, IgM, IgD and IgE do not cross the placental barrier. The mechanism by which the Fc controls transport is not known, but it has been suggested [10, 11] that molecules to be specifically transported are bound to specific receptors on the walls of pinocytotic vacuoles of cells of the placenta and this protects them from degradation and facilitates intercellular transport. This type of mechanism has also been proposed [10, 12] for the regulation of catabolism of immunoglobulins. Binding of IgG to the receptors protects it from degradation – IgG not thus protected is degraded by enzymes and the protected IgG subsequently released. In this way constant levels of IgG are maintained. Again, it appears that the site which regulates immunoglobulin catabolism is also in the Fc region. The metabolism of immunoglobulins has recently been the subject of a detailed review article [13].

Binding of antibodies to macrophages Antibodies are capable of binding to macrophages in the absence of antigen. It seems that such cytophilic binding with macrophage receptors occurs via the Fc region of the antibody. Immune adherence of antigen to macrophage could thus be achieved via this cytophilic antibody which is then followed by phagocytosis. It is more likely however, that adherence and phagocytosis are mediated via opsonic antibody. In this case, antibodies (IgG1 and IgG3 subclasses) bind the antigen via their antibody binding sites and binding to the receptors of the macrophages is achieved through the specific Fc binding site. Recent evidence [14] indicates that the monocyte binding site is in the C_H3 region of the IgG.

Reactivity with rheumatoid factors Rheumatoid factors (RF) are anti-immunoglobulin antibodies which react with various antigenic determinants of human IgG. Such antibodies are found in the sera of patients with rheumatoid arthritis and other conditions. It has been suggested that conformational alteration of the IgG molecule either by aggregation or reaction with antibody results in the formation of sites in the Fc with which RF can react. However, RF also react with native IgG. Genetic antigens (Gm markers) (see Table 3.3) are frequently involved in RF reactions and these Fc antigenic specificities have been partially localized, using proteolytic fragments of human IgG subclasses [5]. Two such sites have been demonstrated in the pFc subfragment of IgG (the C_H3 homology region) and three further sites have been localised in the C_H2 region. The relative importance of the reaction of RF with native and aggregated IgG is the subject of considerable debate [16. 17].

References

[1] Stanworth, D.R. & Turner, M.W. (1973), in *Handbook of Experimental Immunology*,

(D.M. Weir, Ed) 2nd edition, Blackwell Scientific Publications, Oxford, page 10, Vol. 1.

[2] Tomasi, T.B. & Bienenstock, J. (1968), *Advanc. Immunol.* **9**, 1.

[3] Stanworth, D.R. (1973) *Immediate hypersensitivity*, Frontiers of Biology, North-Holland, London & Amsterdam, Volume **28**.

[4] Müller-Eberhard, H.J. (1971), in *Progress in Immunology*, Vol. 1. (Ed. B. Amos), Academic Press, New York and London, p. 553.

[5] Lachmann, P.J., Hobart, M.J. & Aston, W.P. (1973), in *Handbook of Experimental Immunology*, (D.M. Weir, Ed.) 2nd Edition, Blackwell Scientific Publications, Oxford, page 5, Vol. 1.

[6] Gotze, O. & Muller-Eberhard, H.J. (1971), *J. Exp. Med.* **134**, 90.

[7] Müller-Eberhard, H.J. (1968), *Advanc. Immunol.* **8**, 2.

[8] Müller-Eberhard, H.J. (1969), *Ann. Rev. Biochem.* **38**, 389.

[9] Lachmann, P.J. (1973), in *Clinical Aspects of Immunology*, (Gell, P.G.H. & Coombs, R.R.A., Eds.), 3rd edition, Blackwell Scientific Publications, Oxford.

[10] Brambell, F.W.R., Halliday, R. & Hemmings, W.A. (1958), *Proc. Roy. Soc. B.* **149**, 1.

[11] Brambell, F.W.R. (1966), *Lancet*, **2**, 1087.

[12] Brambell, F.W.R., Hemmings, W.A. & Morris, I.G. (1964), *Nature*, **203**, 1352.

[13] Waldmann, T.A. & Strober, W., (1969). *Progr. Allergy*, **13**, 1.

[14] Okafor, G., Hay, F.C. & Turner, M.W. (1973), Personal communication.

[15] Natvig. J.B., Gaarder, P.I. & Turner, M.W. (1972), *Clin. Exp. Immunol.* **12**, 177.

[16] Normansell, D.E. (1971), *Immunochemistry*, **8**, 593.

[17] Roitt, I.M. (1971), *Progress in Immunology*, **1** (B. Amos, Ed), p. 689, Academic Press, New York and London.

Suggestions for further reading

A. Introductory books

Roitt, I.M. (1971), *Essential Immunology*, Blackwell Scientific Publications, Oxford.

Humphrey, J.H. & White, R.G. (1970), *Immunology for Students of Medicine* 3rd edition, Blackwell Scientific Publications, Oxford.

Both these books are excellent introductory texts to the whole field of immunology.

B. Advanced books

Borek, F. Ed. (1972), *Immunogenicity – physicochemical and biological aspects*, Frontiers of Biology, Volume 25. North Holland, Amsterdam and London.

A comprehensive book containing articles by leading workers in the field.

Williams, C.A. and Chase, M.W. Eds. (1967–1971), *Methods of Immunology and Immunochemistry*, Volumes I–IV, Academic Press, New York and London.

Weir, D.M., Ed. (1973), *Handbook of Experimental Immunology*, Blackwell Scientific Publications, Oxford.

These books cover all the modern experimental approaches to immunology.

Antibodies Cold Spring Harbor Symposium on Quantitative Biology (1967).

An historically important book in the development of immunology containing original papers presented at the Symposium in 1967.

Immunoglobulins Annals of the New York Academy of Science (1971) Volume 190.

Contains papers presented at the Academy in December 1971 and is therefore quite up to date.

Day, E.D. (1972) *Advanced Immunochemistry*, Williams and Wilkins, Baltimore.

Particularly good for its discussion of antibody: antigen reactions.

Fudenberg, H.H., Pink, J.L.R., Stites, D.P. and Wang, A-C, (1972), *Basic Immunogenetics*, Oxford University Press, Oxford.

A comprehensive and readable treatment of a complex field.

Index